PREVENTING CERVI

WHAT EVERY WOM

PREVENTING CERVICAL CANCER
WHAT EVERY WOMAN SHOULD KNOW

Anne Szarewski MBBS DRCOG PhD FFFP
Clinical Consultant, Honorary Senior Lecturer, Cancer Research UK
Centre for Epidemiology, Mathematics and Statistics, Wolfson Institute
of Preventive Medicine, London

ALTMAN

Published by Altman Publishing, 7 Ash Copse, Bricket Wood, St Albans, Herts, AL2 3YA

First edition 2007

Typeset in 10/12 Optima by Phoenix Photosetting, Chatham, Kent
Printed in Great Britain by Chiltern Printers (Slough) Ltd

ISBN13: 978-1-86036-042-8

A catalogue record for this book is available from the British Library

∞ Printed on acid-free text paper, manufactured in accordance with
ANSI/NISO Z39.48-1992 (Permanence of Paper)

CONTENTS

PREFACE

Every year in this country hundreds of thousands of women have an abnormal smear. Around three thousand are told the sad news that they have cervical cancer, and roughly half of those women will die of the disease. Most of those deaths could be prevented by adequate screening and treatment. However, many women still do not go for cervical smears because they are frightened or do not understand the importance of the test. Those who do have a smear and are then told it is abnormal often think the worst, again through lack of knowledge and understanding.

The majority of women I have seen, both for smears and for colposcopy, have only a vague idea of what the tests are for, what they mean and what can be done if something is wrong. They want information but have often found it difficult to obtain. Then again, they may have read or been told certain things that are no longer thought to be true. This area of medicine has been changing rapidly and opinions thought to have been correct a few years ago are not necessarily so now. Indeed, it is almost inevitable that some of the information presented in this book will be out of date within a short time of its publication.

It is frustrating that there are still many unanswered or only partially answered questions in this field. We all find it difficult to deal with uncertainty. In this book I have not tried to give simple answers; where there are areas of doubt, I have stated them and presented the arguments for each point of view. I have tried to do this fairly, but inevitably my own biases will have crept in occasionally. I should make the point that the views I express in this book are mine and may not necessarily represent those of Cancer Research UK. In many cases this is because I am writing for you as an individual, and what is best for an individual may not always be applicable to, or indeed appropriate for, society as a whole.

Clinics are busy places and women often feel they cannot ask questions, or that the doctor will not have time to talk to them. Frequently, when faced with a doctor, women forget everything they wanted to ask anyway. I hope that a book such as this will provide information in a non-threatening way and then give you the confidence to ask questions that are specifically related to you, and that cannot be answered properly by any book or leaflet. Although I am sure the majority of readers will be women, it should not be forgotten that men are also involved, and may be worried for their partners: I hope this book will be of use to some of them, too.

I would like to thank Maggie Raynor for line drawings taken from Szarewski, A. *A Woman's Guide to the Cervical Smear Test*, London: Optima, 1994; Louise Cadman, my research nurse consultant and a nurse colposcopist, for taking the time to read through the text and making constructive comments. Any errors that remain are entirely mine.

I would also like to thank my editor and publisher, Peter Altman, for his encouragement and enthusiasm.

AS

1 WHAT IS THE CERVIX? WHAT IS A SMEAR?

The cervix is part of the womb, or uterus. Figure 1.1 shows where the womb sits in the pelvis. You will see that it is connected to the ovaries by a pair of tubes, called the Fallopian tubes (after an Italian doctor called Fallopio). Eggs produced in the ovaries travel down these tubes in order to reach the womb. If you think of the womb as being like an upside-down pear, the cervix is the lower, narrower part. The womb is really just

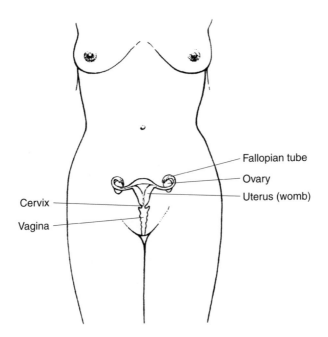

Figure 1.1   Female reproductive organs.

a box designed to contain a baby. The upper part, called the 'body' of the uterus, is where the baby is held and nourished when a woman is pregnant; it expands greatly during pregnancy as the baby gets bigger. The cervix, on the other hand, does not expand much until labour starts. Then it has to open up quickly, to let the baby out.

Both the body of the uterus and the cervix are made of muscle; the body of the uterus needs strong muscle tissue to push a baby out. Unfortunately, these strong muscles are also responsible for period cramps, which can be very painful in some women. The cervix also needs strong muscle, but for the opposite reason – to keep the growing, heavy baby in the womb until it is ready to come out. The cervix has two main muscle areas, called the internal os and the external os (see Figure 1.2).

The muscle around the internal os is the innermost and strongest; it is the one primarily responsible for making sure the baby stays where it should. The external os, as its name suggests, is on the outside. Seen face on, the external os is a hole; in a woman who has not had children, or who has had them by Caesarean section, the hole is small, round and tight (see Figure 1.3). However, during childbirth, when the baby has to pass through it, the hole is stretched a great deal and does not return to its original shape and size. Instead, it becomes slit-shaped and wider than before.

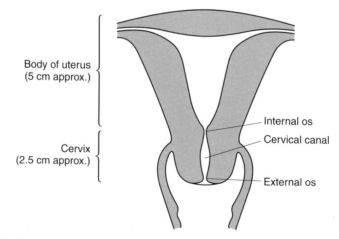

Body of uterus
(5 cm approx.)

Cervix
(2.5 cm approx.)

Internal os

Cervical canal

External os

Figure 1.2 Uterus and cervix.

2

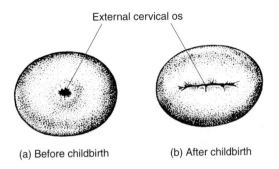

External cervical os

(a) Before childbirth   (b) After childbirth

Figure 1.3   View of the cervix, face on.

Not only babies pass through the hole in the cervix; this is where the blood comes out when you have a period. Sperm use it to gain entry to the womb. If you have an intrauterine device (IUD) fitted for contraception, it has to be pushed past the muscles of both the external os and the internal os, neither of which take too kindly to the idea – this is what can make the procedure uncomfortable. Unpleasant things such as infections can also creep in this way.

The cervix under a magnifying glass

Actually, we need more than a magnifying glass, we need to look through a microscope. This gives even more magnification, so that we can see the individual building blocks, or cells, from which the cervix is made.

All the tissues in the body are made up of different types of cells. Cells are a little like fabrics: some are very delicate and fine, some are stronger and coarser. Just as we use delicate fabrics for clothes and strong ones for upholstery, so cells have different functions, too.

The body of the uterus is lined with soft, columnar (tall and narrow, like columns) cells (see Figure 1.4). They are responsible for providing a growing pregnancy with nourishment; this has to arrive via blood vessels, so these cells have a good blood supply. The lining builds up each month in preparation for a possible pregnancy, but if none occurs, it comes off, bleeding while it does so. This is what you know as a period.

Meanwhile, the cells on the outside surface of both the cervix and the vagina (front passage) have a much harder life. They are like the 'front line' protecting the body of the womb from the outside world. They may

3

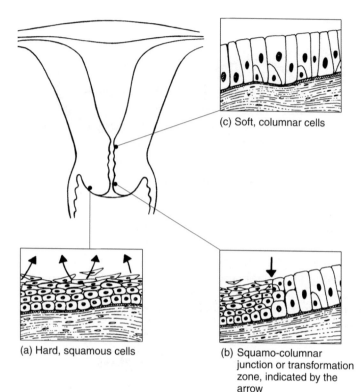

(c) Soft, columnar cells

(a) Hard, squamous cells

(b) Squamo-columnar junction or transformation zone, indicated by the arrow

Figure 1.4 Cells of the cervix and uterus.

be bombarded with infections and they must also withstand being hit repeatedly during sex, so they are hard, squamous (meaning flat) cells. They don't have such a good blood supply – otherwise they would bleed every time you made love.

Of course, there has to be a point at which the two types of cell (squamous and columnar) meet, since the body of the uterus (womb) and the cervix are not actually physically separated from one another. And indeed, this area is called the squamo-columnar junction. In this area, soft columnar cells gradually change to become harder, squamous cells. Cells which are preoccupied with internal changes are more vulnerable to outside attack, so we will be looking at this area again in Chapter 2, when we discuss how abnormal cells appear.

The outside layers of cells are separated from the deeper (known as 'connective') tissues containing blood vessels and glands by a continuous layer of cells called the basement membrane (see Figure 1.5). This acts as a physical barrier and will be very important when we discuss the development of invasive cancer in Chapter 6.

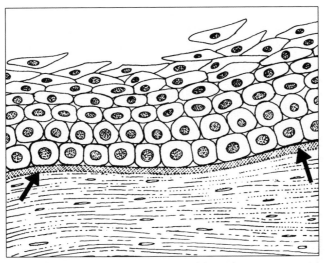

Figure 1.5 Squamous layer of cells separated from the connective tissue by the basement membrane.

When seen under a microscope, the surface of the cervix is not smooth, but has many tiny folds, rather like the irregular pattern of a coastline. The 'bays' are called crypts and, if they become blocked off, they form little fluid-filled cysts, rather like a lagoon that becomes a lake. They can be seen and sometimes felt as little 'bumps' on the surface of the cervix and are called Nabothian follicles, after the doctor who first described them.

What is a cervical smear? What does having one involve?

A cervical smear is a simple screening test for early changes in the cells which may lead to cervical cancer. Cervical cancer is unusual in being theoretically totally preventable by screening, because these early changes can be picked up long before a proper cancer will ever develop. Despite this, around 1500 women die of cervical cancer in the UK every year, many of them because they have not taken up the opportunity to have a smear.

It is important to realise that the test is not looking primarily for proper cancer cells. If that was all it could pick up, it would be a waste of everyone's time – including yours – because many women would still die. The whole point of the test is that the early changes are not actually cancer and are completely curable. Indeed, the definition of a screening test is that it should be done when you are completely well, *before* you have noticed any symptoms.

Any woman who has *ever* had sex should have regular smears. Although cervical cancer can very rarely occur in virgins, it is usually found in women who are or have been sexually active. I shall be discussing the possible causes of cervical cancer in Chapters 7 and 8, so will not dwell on them further here.

What is the examination like?

I was terrified when I went in, but I knew I should try and relax. I kept saying to myself 'relax, relax' but it was impossible. I was afraid of what was going to happen.

A cervical smear involves a vaginal examination. Unfortunately, there is just no other way. So, you will be asked to lie down on a couch, having removed your panties. Your feet will be facing towards a light, which will be used to illuminate your vagina (front passage). The doctor or nurse will need to use an instrument called a speculum to gently hold apart the sides of your vagina, in order to be able to see your cervix. The speculum can be made of metal or plastic (see Figure 1.6) and the two halves will be closed together while it is being inserted, and then they will be opened up once the instrument is inside.

If the speculum is made of metal, its natural state will be freezing cold. Doctors and nurses can forget this, so remind them! The instrument can so easily be warmed by putting it under the hot tap or keeping it on a warm radiator. It is a very small thing, but it will make it a lot easier for you to relax and the whole process becomes simpler.

Did I mention the word 'relax'? Well, difficult though it is, you should try. The more tense you are, the more difficult it will be to open the

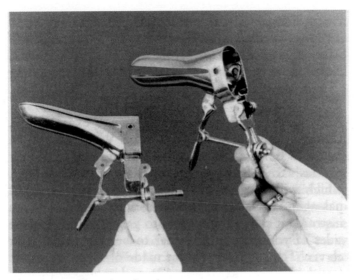

Figure 1.6 A speculum, closed and open.

speculum (after all, you will be positively pushing against it) and the more uncomfortable it will feel. How can you relax? Well, for a start, try not to arrange to have your smear on a day you have an important meeting at work, or are going to be under stress for other reasons. Bring a friend with you, perhaps, at least to sit with in the waiting room.

It is very important that the person taking the smear can get a good view of your cervix; a sample from the wrong place will be of no use and will only result in you having to go through it all again.

Once the cervix is in view, a spatula is gently wiped across it in order to collect some loose cells. Nowadays there is a bewildering variety of instruments that can be used to take smears, ranging from wooden spatulas to nylon brushes. We discuss these in more detail in Chapter 3.

Once the smear has been taken, the speculum is removed and, from your point of view, the procedure is over. You will find, perhaps to your surprise, that the entire event has taken less than 5 minutes.

I expected it to be so much worse. My sister said it was really painful.

I was so embarrassed that he was a man. I hadn't thought about that before at all. It was different when I just had the measles.

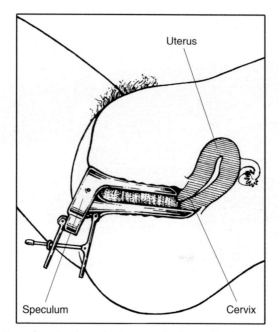

Figure 1.7   Speculum in place during a vaginal examination.

Many women are frightened of having a smear because they don't actually know what it will involve, or, even worse, a friend has had a bad experience and has kindly passed all the details on. I have heard awful stories of rough examinations and unsympathetic doctors or nurses. But they are still in a minority.

> I was in such a state, I was shaking. I was still determined to try and have it done. But when I went in to the nurse, she just talked to me for a few minutes, explaining what the examination involved. Then she gave me leaflet to read. She said I should come back another day, when I'd read the information. She suggested I bring a friend with me as well. I did go back the following week and brought my sister with me. She made me have a gin and tonic before we went in to the clinic! I felt much better and it was OK.

If you are extremely worried, mention this to the doctor or nurse at the start of the appointment. In some cases, they may suggest that you return

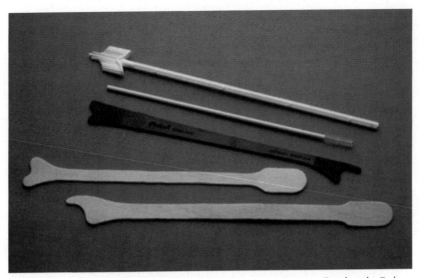

Figure 1.8 Instruments for taking a smear, from top: Cervex, Cytobrush, Rolon spatula, Ayre spatula, Aylesbury spatula.

another day, bringing a friend, or even giving you a mild tranquilliser. One bad experience can make future examinations ten times more difficult, so it is worth making sure you are as prepared as possible. Incidentally, if you have had a traumatic event in the past, such as a rough examination, or if you have been raped and examinations are very emotionally charged, mention it in advance.

If you are uncomfortable with a male doctor, ask for a woman. If there seems to be no choice at your doctor's practice, go to a different one, or to a clinic. You are perfectly entitled to do this, even if you stay with your normal GP for the rest of your care. Incidentally, whether a man or woman takes your smear, you are entitled to ask for a chaperone to be in the room. If you really feel you can't go through with an examination, say so. You can always come back another time. Although smears are for your protection, you shouldn't feel you have been forced to have one. They may be advisable, but they are not compulsory.

Is there a best time to have a smear?

In theory, it is ideal to have a smear taken when you are in the middle of your cycle; the hormonal environment at that time makes the cervix easier to access and the os (opening) is a little wider, allowing an instrument to be inserted more easily into the cervical canal (of course, the real reason for it being wider is to make it easier for sperm to get in while you are at your most fertile).

However, this ideal is taken to the point of silliness. I have seen women who have spent days getting themselves psyched up, turned away, because they did not come exactly mid-cycle. A smear can be done on any day of the month, though preferably not when you are actually bleeding. And if you are using hormonal contraception (e.g. the pill) the whole mid-cycle concept is ridiculous, because you aren't ovulating anyway. So don't allow this mid-cycle idea to put you off; just get it done.

What happens to the smear?

There are now two ways in which the smear may be processed. In the traditional method, the cells are transferred onto a glass slide by wiping the spatula across it. The cells cannot survive for long like this, so they have to be preserved or 'fixed' using an alcohol solution. You may see this being poured onto the slide; sometimes a spray is used instead. Once this has been done, the smear can be kept safely for a long time. It is sent to a laboratory where the cells are stained with various dyes to show up their features more clearly.

There is now a newer technique, called liquid-based cytology (LBC). The difference is that instead of being spread onto a slide, the cells are shaken off into a vial of preservative liquid. For this method, a plastic instrument has to be used, so that the cells come off it successfully; the most common one is called a Cervex, and looks a little like a broom (see Figure 1.9). The vial is then sent off to the laboratory, where the liquid is spun and treated to remove obscuring material, for example blood, mucus or pus, and a random sample of the remaining cells is taken. A thin layer of the cells is then deposited onto a slide and stained in the usual way. The big advantage of this system is that by clearing away blood and mucus, it is much easier to see the cervical cells, which are really important. As a result, you are much less likely to have an unsatisfactory smear and be called back for a repeat.

The cells are examined under a microscope by specially trained technicians and doctors called cytologists. The word 'cytology' simply means 'the study of cells' ('cyto' means 'cell' in Greek, while 'ology' means 'the

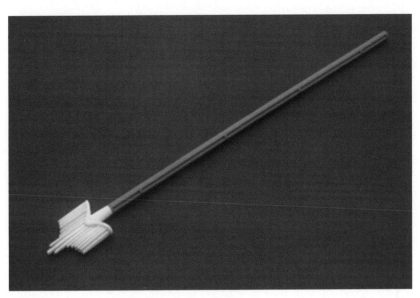

Figure 1.9   Cervex for liquid-based cytology.

study of'). Usually the technicians look at each slide first; any they think may show an abnormality will then be double-checked by a doctor. Although it may take weeks for you to hear the result, during most of that time your slide will be sitting idle in a pile, waiting for its turn. The actual process of checking it takes about 20 minutes on average.

A report will then be sent back to your doctor or clinic. The report may come back on the original smear form, though in some laboratories they now produce computer print-outs. Whichever method is used, the reporting is mostly standardised. Although most women never get to see their smear report, there is actually no reason why this should be so. One of my aims in this book is to explain the report form and the reporting system so that you should be able to understand your own smear result.

The cervical smear form

Figure 1.10 shows the current nationally used smear form. The left hand side is for your personal details, your name, address, date of birth, registration number. Also given are your doctor's name and address. If it is not

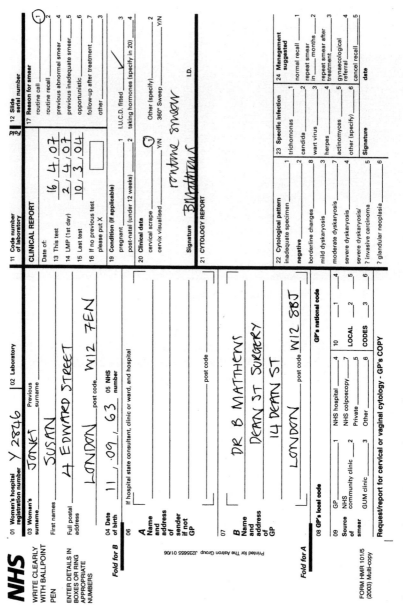

Figure 1.10 The NHS cervical smear form.

12

your GP who is taking the smear, his/her details are given anyway so that they can be sent a copy of the result.

On the right-hand side there are details about your relevant medical history (section 11, see Figure 1.11). The date of the current smear is given and also the date of your last smear. This allows the laboratory to check the time interval between your smears; some laboratories may now reject smears taken at more frequent intervals than they consider appropriate – we discuss this again in Chapter 9. More helpfully, if there is a query about your current result, they may be able to recheck the slide sent to them previously (but only if both were sent to the same laboratory).

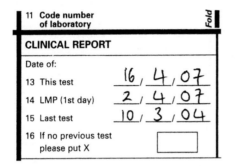

Figure 1.11 Close-up of section 11, dealing with date of test and last menstrual period (LMP).

The date of your last period is important, because the appearance of the cells varies at different times of the menstrual cycle. Cells also look different if you have gone past the change of life (the menopause), so if the date of the last period is several months or years ago, the cytologist will be alerted to the fact that this may be the case.

Section 19 (see Figure 1.12) gives other medical details, for example whether you are pregnant or have recently had a baby (postnatal). An IUD (intrauterine contraceptive device or coil) can also sometimes make

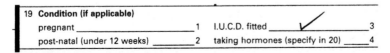

Figure 1.12 Section 19 of the NHS smear form.

the cells look slightly unusual and may result in them being called abnormal if the cytologist is unaware that you have an IUD (the form still uses the old abbreviation IUCD, rather than IUD). Hormones, whether they are being taken for contraceptive, hormone replacement or other reasons, may alter the expected appearance of the cells (particularly since they may not look 'right' for the supposed time of a natural menstrual cycle). More details will then be written in section 20 (see below).

```
17  Reason for smear
     routine call _____(  1  )
     routine recall _____ 2
     previous abnormal smear _____ 4
     previous inadequate smear _____ 5
     opportunistic _____ 6
     follow-up after treatment _____ 7
     other _____ 3
```

Figure 1.13   Section 17 of the NHS smear form.

Section 17 (see Figure 1.13) tells the lab whether this is a routine smear, or whether there is a special reason why you are having one at this time, for example that you have had an abnormal smear in the past, or that the doctor feels you should have one because of abnormal bleeding. It is useful for the laboratory to know if you have been treated for an abnormality ('follow-up after treatment'). Once again, more details will be given in section 20.

Section 20 (see Figure 1.14) contains a blank area for the doctor or nurse to write in anything they feel is relevant. For example, this is where they would specify which type of hormones you were taking. It is also important to know if the smear is being taken from the vagina for some

```
20  Clinical data
     cervical scrape _____( 1 )     Other (specify)_____ 2
     cervix visualised _____ Y/N     360° Sweep _____ Y/N

                    routine smear
     Signature    B Matthews              I.D.
```

Figure 1.14   Section 20 of the NHS smear form with some details filled in.

reason, for example following a hysterectomy, in which case 'other' will be ticked.

The bottom left-hand section (22; see Figure 1.15) gives the smear report. For example, if it is negative, the number 2, opposite 'negative' will be circled. If the sample was inadequate and needs to be repeated, number 1, opposite 'inadequate specimen' will be circled. The rest of the classifications in section 22 are discussed in Chapter 2.

Section 23 (Figure 1.15) is used if any infections were noticed on the smear. For example, if candida (thrush) is picked up on the smear, the number 2 will be circled. Infections are discussed in more detail in Chapter 3.

Section 21 (Figure 1.15) is a blank space where the cytologist can write any extra comments about your smear. Often there will be nothing written in it; however, it is this section that can cause a lot of anxiety and misunderstanding. The most common phrases you are likely to see are 'No endocervical cells seen', 'Endocervical cells seen' and 'Inflammatory changes'. These terms are explained in Chapter 3. It is not unknown for the comments to be so technical that other doctors cannot understand

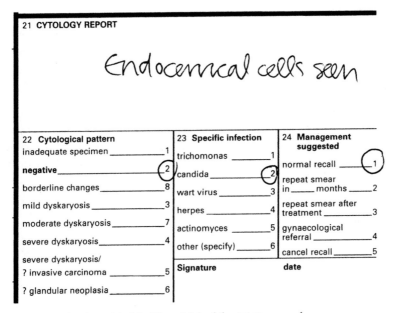

Figure 1.15   Sections 21, 22, 23 and 24 of the NHS smear form.

them either.... Hopefully, this book will make at least the more common ones less threatening.

In section 24 (Figure 1.15) the cytologist recommends what course of action should be taken following this smear. For example, if it is negative, they will tick 'normal recall'. The actual timing of your next smear will depend on what 'normal recall' is in your area; it varies according to government guidelines, local resources and doctors' opinions (not necessarily in that order). This is discussed fully in Chapter 9. If you need further investigations, number 4 ('gynaecological referral') will be ticked or circled. Sometimes an infection has obscured the smear and a repeat will be required after the infection has been treated; in this case number 3 will be circled.

Your doctor may choose not to follow the recommendation given on the smear form; it is, after all, only 'management suggested'. If there is a discrepancy, or if you are unsure of what is happening, ask for an explanation, don't just go home and worry about it.

Obviously, the most important part of the form is section 22, which tells you whether your smear is negative or not. Let us now look at the meaning of the phrase 'positive smear'.

2 WHAT IS AN ABNORMAL SMEAR?

I opened the envelope and there it was: my smear was positive. I was going to die. Why me? What had I done? I burst into tears.

There was a long letter and an information sheet, explaining all about cell changes. The words swam in front of my eyes, I felt dizzy. All I could think about were those two words 'positive smear'.

The term 'abnormal' or 'positive smear' must be one of the most emotive in medicine. And yet, all it is referring to is a smear which is not normal or negative. The term encompasses every grade of abnormality, from borderline abnormal cells right through to cancer. Why do so many women immediately assume the worst? In the UK there are probably about 300 000 abnormal smear results every year. And yet the number of women who are found to have cancer is about 3000, of whom many have not had a smear at all. So an abnormal smear result is very, very, very unlikely to mean you have cancer. But what *does* it mean?

Abnormal cell changes

Chapter 1 looked at the different types of cells, or building blocks, which make up the cervix. You may remember that there are two types, the soft columnar ones and the hard, squamous ones. Where soft columnar cells are exposed to the outside world, they gradually adapt by changing into tougher squamous cells. This happens around the area of the cervical canal and is called the squamo-columnar junction. The process, which is quite normal, is called squamous metaplasia (metaplasia means change, or transformation). The area in which this change, or transformation, takes place is also called the transformation zone (see Figure 2.1).

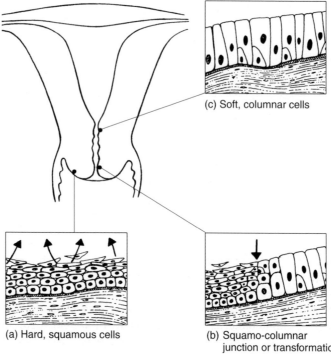

(c) Soft, columnar cells

(a) Hard, squamous cells

(b) Squamo-columnar junction or transformation zone, indicated by the arrow

Figure 2.1   Cells of the cervix and uterus.

Cells which are changing are occupied and 'off guard'. Thus, it is these cells that are the ones most vulnerable to attack; they may start to change in the 'wrong' way and, if so, eventually could become cancer cells.

These changes do not occur overnight; in fact, it is a very slow process. It has been estimated that it probably takes around 10 years for normal cells to become cancer cells.

Cells that are starting to change abnormally can be distinguished from normal ones under the microscope. They tend to be smaller and have a larger nucleus relative to the rest of the cell. The nucleus is like a brain directing the cell, telling it what to do. Figure 2.2 will give you an idea of the different appearances of normal and abnormal cells.

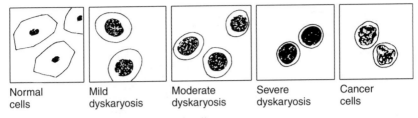

| Normal cells | Mild dyskaryosis | Moderate dyskaryosis | Severe dyskaryosis | Cancer cells |

Figure 2.2   Normal and abnormal cells.

There are a couple of different terms used to describe cells that are changing abnormally. The oldest, 'dysplasia' comes from the Greek 'dys' which means 'bad' or 'abnormal' and 'plasia' which means change, i.e. abnormal change. Thus 'mild dysplasia' means 'mild abnormal change', 'moderate dysplasia' means a 'moderately abnormal change', 'severe dysplasia' means 'severely abnormal change'. They represent increasingly abnormal stages of change in the cells, but none of them is cancer.

Another terminology, which is used in the UK, is 'dyskaryosis' (see Figure 2.3). Once again, 'dys' means 'bad' or 'abnormal'; the word 'karyon' means 'nucleus'. This terminology therefore emphasises the changes that occur in the nucleus of the cell. Nevertheless, it is synonymous with dysplasia, so 'mild dyskaryosis' is equivalent to 'mild dysplasia', 'moderate dyskaryosis' to 'moderate dysplasia' and 'severe dyskaryosis' to 'severe dysplasia'. Most other countries still use the term 'dysplasia', so you may easily come across both.

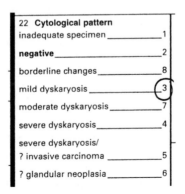

Figure 2.3   Section 22 of NHS smear form.

19

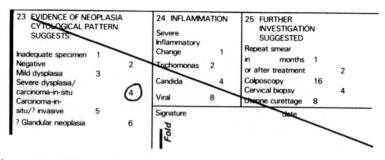

23 EVIDENCE OF NEOPLASIA CYTOLOGICAL PATTERN SUGGESTS:		24 INFLAMMATION		25 FURTHER INVESTIGATION SUGGESTED	
		Severe Inflammatory Change	1	Repeat smear	
Inadequate specimen	1			in months	1
Negative	2	Trichomonas	2	or after treatment	2
Mild dysplasia	3			Colposcopy	16
Severe dysplasia/ carcinoma-in-situ	(4)	Candida	4	Cervical biopsy	4
Carcinoma-in- situ/? invasive	5	Viral	8	Uterine curettage	8
? Glandular neoplasia	6	Signature		date	
		Fold			

Figure 2.4 Old smear form showing 'carcinoma-in situ'.

If you see an old smear form (Figure 2.4), you may notice the term 'carcinoma-in-situ'. This sounds awful (the Latin 'in situ' means 'which has not spread', i.e. 'cancer that has not spread'); however it still means severe dysplasia or severe dyskaryosis, but where the cytologist felt it might soon become cancer. This term has been withdrawn because it caused a great deal of anxiety and confusion. However, in order to allow a cytologist to differentiate between 'severe dyskaryosis – not too much to worry about' and 'severe dyskaryosis – hurry up and investigate', they have introduced the category 'severe dyskaryosis/?invasive cancer' (see Figure 2.3).

Please don't allow these complicated arguments to obscure the main point of all this. Cells that are changing abnormally are **absolutely not** cancer until they move on a stage from severe dyskaryosis. And indeed, many of them will never become cancer. The whole beauty of the smear test is that the cells can be identified when they are still completely harmless; they have the potential to become cancer in some women, but won't do so for a long time, if at all. Thus they, and any chance of cancer, can be removed easily and well in time.

Yet another classification system – CIN

I'm afraid so. Just as you thought you'd got it sorted out in your mind, here is another terminology. However, this one is not so different from the others, only it doesn't refer to individual cells, it refers to their arrangement in the cervix.

CIN stands for cervical intra-epithelial neoplasia. If you remember that 'plasia' means 'change', then 'neo' means 'new', i.e. 'new change'.

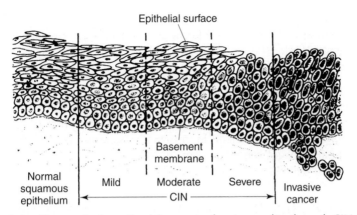

Figure 2.5   Changes in the cells of the cervix, from normality through CIN to an invasive cancer.

'Intra' means 'in' and 'epithelial' refers to the outer layers of cells which act as a protective covering for the blood vessels and glands (known as connective tissues, see Chapter 1). 'Cervical' simply means 'of the cervix'. So CIN means 'new changes occurring in the outer layers of cells of the cervix'.

This classification refers to the way abnormal cells are arranged in the cervix. If only one-third of the thickness of the epithelium (outer layers of skin) is involved, this is the first stage of abnormality, CIN 1. If two-thirds are involved, that is CIN 2. If the whole thickness consists of abnormal cells, that is CIN 3. As you may have realised, this cannot be seen on a smear, because a smear just consists of loose cells. So, to see CIN under the microscope, you need a small piece of the cervix, called a biopsy. This is discussed in more detail in Chapter 4.

In fact, CIN 1 can be thought of as equivalent to 'mild dysplasia/ dyskaryosis', CIN 2 as equivalent to 'moderate dysplasia/dyskaryosis' and CIN 3 as equivalent to 'severe dysplasia/dyskaryosis'.

Because 'CIN' is shorter and quicker to say than 'dyskaryosis' or 'dysplasia', the terms are often used interchangeably. For example, a smear showing 'mild dyskaryosis' may be referred to as a 'CIN 1 smear'. Strictly speaking this is incorrect because, as mentioned above, it is not possible to diagnose CIN from loose cells on a smear. Don't worry about it at present, but I shall return to this concept again later.

21

I was sitting in the surgery and the doctor was trying to explain what was wrong with my smear. I know she said 'cancer', I heard it. I can't understand why she was trying to make it sound less serious. I've got cancer and that's that.

Once again, it is important to stress that, by definition, no grade of CIN is cancer. It has sometimes been called 'pre-cancer' to emphasise the fact that it is 'before cancer', but the term is self-defeating because the very presence of the word 'cancer' in 'pre-cancer' causes a panic. I know this is beginning to get repetitive, but these are just cells which have the *potential* to develop into cancer over a long period of time.

I'm sorry, but there is yet another terminology...

Yes, doctors just can't get enough. This one groups the grades of abnormality into two categories, low grade and high grade. So human papillomavirus (HPV) changes and mild abnormalities become 'low-grade squamous intra-epithelial lesions', or LSIL, while CIN 2, CIN 3 and anything worse become 'high-grade squamous intra-epithelial lesions', or HSIL. Borderline changes become 'abnormal cells of uncertain significance', or ASCUS, to reflect the fact that they really don't mean a lot. Indeed, someone has joked that what it really stands for is 'don't ASK US'. This system is called the Bethesda System, reflecting the fact that it was developed by the American National Cancer Institute, based in Bethesda, Maryland.

I have an abnormal smear, what happens next?

I sat and looked at the letter for 5 days. It just said 'There is no cause for alarm. Please come and discuss your smear result with the doctor at your earliest convenience.' But when I rang the surgery, they said I couldn't be seen for 5 days. I couldn't work, I couldn't sleep, I didn't want to see anyone. I didn't want to tell my family or my friends. I didn't know what to say.

The doctor was very helpful, explained that it wasn't anything serious but I would need to have a special examination. He gave me some leaflets to read and said I could always come back if I had any questions. The information helped a lot, as I was able to read it when I was feeling a little better. I did go back to him and I borrowed a book from the library. I wanted to understand exactly what was going on.

The most common reaction to being informed of an abnormal smear seems to be that of blind panic. Why? Because doctors, health educators, schools, the media have all somehow failed to get across the simple message that an abnormal smear does not mean cancer, that it is just an early warning of something which may - or may not - develop later. Many standard letters also do not give the exact result, they just say the smear is abnormal and you should come and discuss it. This would be fine if you were able to discuss it straight away, but the chances are you will have to wait a few days, imagining the worst all the time. To my mind it is less frightening to know straight away in the letter exactly what is going on – provided some information is included to explain the result. However, the chances are that you will need to see your doctor to find out.

When I got the letter, I was really worried. Only last month my friend Angela was talking about someone who went through all this last year and had a terrible time. There was a mix-up over the results, she wasn't seen when she should have been and in the end she nearly got cancer. She's fine now, but apparently she's very bitter. Angela said she often talks about it.

The next day I went in to work. I hadn't intended to mention it at all, but it just came out, I couldn't stop myself. My boss, Julia, was so sympathetic, she said she'd had an abnormal smear 3 years ago. She told me all about the hospital and the examination I would have to have. It made me feel much better, as she seemed to be quite OK about it. She said it hadn't been nearly as bad as she had expected beforehand and told me not to worry too much.

While you are waiting for your appointment with the doctor, use the delay to prepare yourself. Get as much information as you can, from leaflets, books, organisations. Talk to your friends. You will almost certainly be surprised to find how many women you know who have been through the experience. Around 300 000 women every year in this country have some kind of abnormal smear, so you are certainly not alone. Bear in mind, though, when you talk to friends, that those few who have had bad experiences usually have the most vivid memories. If you hear horror stories, try and find someone who had a better experience, to redress the balance a little.

When you see the doctor, make sure you are told exactly what your smear result was. There is no reason at all why you should not see your own result form. Your doctor may be worried it will frighten you because you won't understand it. However, one of the purposes of this book is precisely to help you understand smear reports, so that you can then understand why you are having investigations and so on. Many women find it more frightening not to be shown the report: after all, why is there something to hide?

Once you have established what grade of abnormality the smear showed, you will need to discuss what is going to happen next. This is very straightforward if the result showed moderate or severe dyskaryosis (or, of course, in the rare event the result suggests cancer); you will be referred to a hospital for colposcopy.

Colposcopy is simply a way of taking a closer look at the cervix through a large magnifying glass, and is described in detail in Chapter 4. There are three important things that happen at colposcopy. The first is that the doctor can, with a good degree of accuracy, tell whether or not you have cancer. The chances are that you won't and so he or she will be able to reassure you about this immediately. If everything looks completely normal, you will also be told that straight away. If there is an abnormal-looking area present, the actual grade of abnormality can be suggested, but not guaranteed to be accurate. For this reason, a tiny piece, or biopsy, will be taken, to be checked in a laboratory. If you recall our discussion of CIN, this little piece of the cervix allows the grade of CIN to be determined.

If colposcopy and biopsy confirm the presence of CIN 2 or 3 (the second or third stage of abnormal cells), it is likely you will be advised to have treatment, and the various options are presented in Chapter 5.

The dilemma of the mildly abnormal smear

Things are not so straightforward if the result is borderline or mild dyskaryosis. This means the cells are only showing borderline or mild abnormalities. Should you have a colposcopy, or should you simply have another smear in 6 months? The medical world is divided over this issue. On the one hand, people argue, mild abnormalities often go away on their own; why investigate straight away, give it time. And even if a mild abnormality is there, nothing is going to happen in 6 months, or even a year. After all, the cell changes occur very slowly, over several years, not

6 or even 12 months. And some women are made more anxious by having to go to the hospital for further investigations; they would be less worried by having a repeat smear. All this is true.

The other argument is this: certainly mild abnormalities are not dangerous and can easily be left alone. But can we be sure that the abnormality really is mild? A number of studies have shown that up to half of smears showing 'mild dyskaryosis' are wrong. When these women have a colposcopy, they are found to have CIN 2 or even CIN 3, despite the smear suggesting only a mild abnormality. The same applies to about a fifth of smears that show borderline changes. So can we be sure it is safe to wait? And some women are made more anxious not knowing exactly what is going on, they would prefer to be investigated. All this is also true.

So what should you, the person in the middle, do? Well, partly it does depend on how you see it. What will make you feel better, having repeat smears, or being investigated? The odds are certainly in favour of the fact that nothing adverse will happen to you, whichever course you choose.

But what about those smears that are wrong, where you already have CIN 2 or 3? This is the main problem, as I see it, and is the reason I tend towards investigation. Even though, as I have said, the odds are in your favour, I dislike uncertainty. Once you *know* you only have CIN 1, fine, don't have it treated; wait and see if it gets better on its own. But you don't know that from the smear, you will have a better idea after a colposcopy and biopsy, when they have looked under the microscope at the arrangement of the cells. In the last few years, the NHS Cervical Screening Programme has also tended towards this view, and has recommended that ideally, women should be referred for colposcopy after one mildly abnormal smear (this does not apply to borderline smears, where both they and I agree it is safe just to repeat the smear). However, they acknowledge that not all areas have the capacity to refer so many women, so it is acceptable to repeat the smear in 6 months. I'm afraid I see this as another postcode lottery and would rather it was the woman who made that decision, allowing her an (informed, of course) choice.

I have suggested that proven CIN 1 does not need treatment: why? Remember that CIN 1 has got to go through CIN 2 and CIN 3 before cancer can develop. It isn't going to do that very fast, it will take years. Sometimes the cells will change back and become normal on their own. Indeed, it has been shown that just taking the tiny biopsy often helps a small area of abnormality improve, perhaps because it stimulates the body's own immune response and helps it fight back. And if it doesn't get better and you go on to develop CIN 2? The treatment is very simple and you are still not in any danger.

Some women prefer to avoid medical intervention and try homeopathy or another type of alternative medicine. This is fine for CIN 1. There is no scientific evidence either way, but, as I have said, watching and waiting at this stage will not do any harm. And it may make you feel you are doing something positive to help yourself.

Incidentally, you may be wondering why CIN 2 or even 3 need treatment, when neither is cancer. The reason is that they seem less likely to go away on their own and may get worse. It could certainly be argued that a small area of CIN 2 could be left a while. But since we do not know the precise time-scale of cell changes, if CIN 3 is there already, it might just tip over into early cancer if left too long.

Does CIN 1 ever need treatment? Yes, sometimes. The most important reason is if you feel too anxious about leaving it, even after reading this book. But make sure you have considered what the treatment involves, simple though it is; read Chapter 5. The second reason is if the area involved is large, because it is less likely to get better on its own. Also, if it becomes even larger, it may become technically difficult to treat, should the cells move on to CIN 2 or 3. In such a case, although there is no hard and fast rule, I often feel it would be better to treat sooner rather than later. Another reason to favour treatment is if you will not be able to return for monitoring. Say you have a job which takes you around the world for long periods of time, or you are going to emigrate somewhere where the medical facilities may be poor – then you might just prefer to be treated and get the whole thing over and done with.

Of course, what I have described is an ideal. As already mentioned, you may not be offered a choice between repeat smears or immediate colposcopy at all. Financial constraints have meant that in many areas you will not be offered a colposcopy after one mildly abnormal smear. Interestingly, there is now conflicting evidence about the cost of each approach. For a number of years it has been argued that it is cheaper to repeat smears before referral, but recently it has been suggested that by the time a woman has had several repeat smears, possibly ending up with colposcopy anyway, it would actually be cheaper to offer colposcopy straight away!

So, again, what should you do? I do not think it is unreasonable to have a borderline smear repeated 6 months later. Current guidelines say you should have three borderline smears before you are referred for colposcopy, and I don't think this is unreasonable. However, if the smear shows mild dyskaryosis, I would be happier to do a colposcopy after the first abnormal smear.

What if this is impossible in your area? Well, you can ask your GP to refer you somewhere else. Policies are very variable and you may find that a clinic in another district will see you, even if you have to wait a couple of months. Since all you were going to have was a repeat smear in 6 months, even if it takes that long to have the colposcopy, you are still better off. And nothing is likely to happen to you in such a short time; keep reminding yourself that cell changes occur very slowly.

The obvious solution to all these problems would be a way of being able to differentiate (without resorting to colposcopy) between those women who really do only have a mild abnormality and could wait, from those who need to be investigated now. There is a new form of testing, which may help do that, and is discussed further in Chapters 8 and 11.

I had had two smears which showed abnormal cells. When I went to the doctor, I was already psyched up to the idea of a hospital appointment. I'd read about colposcopy and I was prepared for it. I was completely thrown when he said I was going to have to have another smear, again in 6 months' time. Apparently, the waiting list couldn't cope if everyone was seen sooner. I went home, but I was upset. Then I got angry. My health was more important than a stupid waiting list. My first thought was 'I'll go private', and I even rang up a doctor recommended by a friend. It would cost me nearly £300. I don't have insurance and I'm not made of money. Peter said he'd find the money, that of course I should have the best. But I sat down and thought about it again. I decided to go back to the doctor. I was ready for a fight, but he immediately said 'I can see you're upset'. I burst into tears, I couldn't help it. He said he'd do his best to get me an appointment; one of the consultants at another hospital was able to squeeze people in sometimes. It was quite a lot further away, would I mind? Actually, the hospital wasn't far from where Peter works, so it was better in a way. Two months later I went for my appointment. Peter took the afternoon off and came with me. It was a good thing he did; it turned out that I already had CIN 3, much more serious than my smear showed. The consultant booked me in for treatment and it was all got rid of in time. But it's not right I had to fight to be seen. What about women who are frightened of making a fuss?

The doctor explained that when a smear just showed borderline changes, it might sometimes be a mistake, or the changes would go back to normal on their own. When she told me that it depended on people looking down microscopes, trying to decide whether things looked completely normal or not, I could see it might be difficult. She suggested I have a repeat smear in 6 months first. I was happy with that, the hospital appointment seemed a bit frightening, especially if it might not be necessary. My next smear was OK, I was so relieved. The doctor said I'd better have another one in 6 months, just to be sure. That was normal as well. I'm glad it was all so easy in the end.

Glandular abnormalities

You may have a smear result where the last item in Section 22 is highlighted '?glandular neoplasia' (Figure 2.6). In Chapter 1, I mentioned that there are two types of cells in the cervix, the flat squamous cells, and the tall, columnar, endocervical cells. The word 'glandular' refers to the columnar cells. If you have a smear showing ?glandular neoplasia, you will be referred for colposcopy straight away. The reason is that these abnormalities are much more difficult to assess and therefore any suggestion they could be present should be properly investigated. Having said that, in the majority of cases, it turns out there was nothing wrong, or only a very minor abnormality. However, sometimes it will be necessary to perform a loop treatment (see Chapter 5) to be sure.

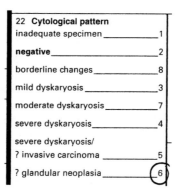

Figure 2.6   Section 22 of NHS smear form, showing '?glandular neoplasia'.

The unsatisfactory, or inadequate smear

The very first heading in section 22 of the smear form is 'inadequate specimen' (Figure 2.7). And it means just what it says – that the smear was not adequate for assessment, and therefore needs to be repeated. You will usually be asked to come back 2–3 months later for a repeat test. Unfortunately, many women think that this is some kind of smokescreen for saying 'we think it's abnormal, but we are not sure, so we're going to do another one' and get themselves very worked up. A recent study showed that women who had an unsatisfactory result were as anxious as those who had been told their smear was abnormal. This is really sad, as no-one is trying to hide anything. If you think about it, the category which covers 'we're not sure if this is really abnormal or not' is the borderline smear.

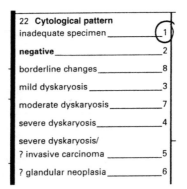

Figure 2.7   Section 22 of NHS smear form, showing 'inadequate specimen'.

Why are smears inadequate for assessment? There may be too few cells on the slide, so whoever took the sample perhaps didn't scrape the cervix properly, or didn't transfer the cells efficiently to the slide. Or there may have been blood or mucus, which has covered the cells and made it impossible to see them. I have never yet seen 'slide dropped on the floor of the laboratory' given as a reason, but I would have thought that was possible as well! Between 5 and 10% of smear samples are unsatisfactory for one of these reasons. The good news is that one of the big advantages of liquid-based cytology (LBC), which is being introduced throughout the UK, is that there are far fewer unsatisfactory smears.

29

Studies have suggested that only around 2% of LBC samples cannot be assessed. There are various reasons for this:

- shaking the instrument into a liquid is a more efficient way of transferring the cells, so the smear is less likely to have too few cells for assessment;
- the processing of the liquid sample effectively means that the cells are 'washed' and blood and mucus removed, again making the smear easier to read.

So it is likely that there will be fewer unsatisfactory smears in the future. Meanwhile, please try not to worry if you receive this result; it really does only mean what it says.

3 WHAT DOES THIS MEAN? A LOOK AT SOME TECHNICAL TERMS

No Endocervical cells seen. Negative

Alternatively, you may see 'Endocervical cells seen. Negative'. Whichever way round it is put, the result seems to be anxiety.

I thought, what are these things they've seen? Why have I got them?

Does that mean my smear is no good? What didn't they see? Will I have to have another one?

---

21 CYTOLOGY REPORT

No endocervical cell seen

22 Cytological pattern	23 Specific infection	24 Management suggested
inadequate specimen _____1	trichomonas _____1	
negative_____(2)	candida _____2	normal recall _____1
borderline changes_____8	wart virus _____3	repeat smear in _____ months _____2
mild dyskaryosis_____3	herpes _____4	repeat smear after treatment _____3
moderate dyskaryosis_____7	actinomyces _____5	gynaecological referral _____4
severe dyskaryosis_____4	other (specify) _____6	cancel recall_____5
severe dyskaryosis/ ? invasive carcinoma _____5	**Signature** **date**	
? glandular neoplasia_____6		

Figure 3.1   Smear form results: negative.

Endocervical cells are similar to the soft, columnar cells which are normally found lining the inside of the womb. They are present at the junction point, called the squamo-columnar junction, where some of them start to change into flat squamous cells. Chapter 2 discussed the importance of this area, since it is the place where abnormal changes are likely to begin.

If this area is important, it would be nice to know that it has been checked by the smear. One of the ways in which we can tell it has been checked is to see endocervical cells. Other markers are columnar cells that are undergoing squamous metaplasia (i.e. that have started the process of changing into flat, squamous cells). They look subtly different from endocervical cells, but are also present at the squamo-columnar junction. Cervical mucus can also be seen on a smear, and is another indicator that the squamo-columnar junction has been checked. In practice, if cytologists see any of these three markers, they may just note 'endocervical cells seen' on the form. However, they may have a policy of only commenting on their absence, rather than their presence.

You would not believe the arguments that have been going on for years about the importance (or otherwise) of seeing squamo-columnar junction markers (which I shall also refer to collectively as endocervical cells from now on). The argument goes like this: if endocervical cells are so important, then we should be able to show that smears that have them are more likely to also be reported as abnormal when there is an abnormal area on the cervix. Alternatively, we should be able to show that smears without endocervical cells are more likely to be falsely reassuring, that the woman has an abnormal area on her cervix, but it has been missed. This second option is impractical, because every woman having a smear would also have to have a colposcopy at the same time (see Chapter 4).

So, we are left with studies that look at different ways of taking smears, comparing abnormality rates with the pick-up of endocervical cells.

Figure 3.2 shows a selection of instruments that have all been designed to take smears. You may also want to look back at Figure 1.8 of Chapter 1. The traditional Ayre spatula has gradually been replaced in the UK by the Aylesbury, which is more pointed. The idea of the point is to try and reach the squamo-columnar junction even if it is not on the outside surface of the cervix, but further up inside the cervical canal (this is more likely in slightly older women, over the age of 35). The Jordan/Rolon spatula, the Cervex and the Cytobrush are further refinements on

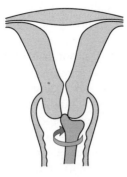

(a) Ayre spatula

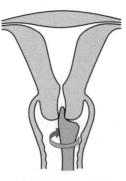

(b) Aylesbury spatula

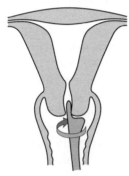

(c) Jordan/Rolon spatula

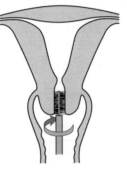

(d) Cytobrush

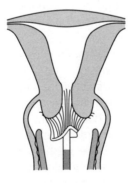

(e) Cervex

Figure 3.2 Instruments designed to take smears.

this idea. The Cervex is the instrument usually used for liquid-based cytology; the idea is that the longer central 'fronds' go into the cervical canal, while the shorter, outer ones sweep over the outer surface of the cervix. The Cytobrush should be used as well as, not instead of, a spatula, because on its own it doesn't sample the outside surface of the cervix at all. This is the ultimate belt and braces approach, covering every possible place where the squamo-columnar junction could be. And, indeed, many studies have shown that if you are interested in endocervical cells, the Cytobrush plus spatula (which must be plastic for liquid-based cytology) combination picks up cells that other methods just cannot reach.

The difficulty is proving that it matters. Logically, from our previous discussion about the squamo-columnar junction, it should make a difference. You should find that you pick up more abnormalities when the smears show the presence of endocervical cells. And indeed, a recent pooling together of a number of studies has shown just that. But there are studies that don't, and therein lies the problem. In many countries, doctors have decided that, until there is conclusive proof it is *not* important, they will do their best to pick up endocervical cells. In this country, the opposite view has generally prevailed, i.e. that until it is conclusively proven that it *does* make a difference, it will not be considered important.

As a result, many laboratories have not been reporting whether endocervical cells are present or not. It must be said that part of the argument in this country is financial; if it is decided that endocervical cells are important, smears not containing them would have to be labelled as inadequate. Women would then have to be recalled for repeat smears and this could involve around 20 or even 30% of the smears taken and therefore a lot of time and money.

In my view, the evidence points to the presence of endocervical cells being important. But there is another, very good reason for reporting endocervical cells: quality control.

Cells from the outside surface of the cervix are very similar (in fact pretty well identical) to those from the vagina: they are all flat, squamous cells. So, if a smear does not contain any of the markers of the squamo-columnar junction (referred to collectively as endocervical cells), it could have been taken from anywhere in the vagina, it may not even have included the cervix at all. The laboratory will simply not be able to tell the difference. In 1993, a nurse in a general practice surgery was found to be using a tongue depressor to take smears. She was apparently doing this for nearly 2 years before it came to light and over a thousand women were asked to have another smear. It is likely that many of the smears she had taken would not have contained endocervical cells; if someone had thought to enquire why this was, she might have been discovered earlier.

Personally, I think this is a really important issue. Even if you train doctors and nurses to take smears, you cannot guarantee that they will all be good at it. Some may have been competent to start with, but may now be 'rusty' due to lack of practice. Others may just be careless. In practical terms, the only way to ensure that smears are being taken correctly is to check whether a doctor or nurse has a particularly high 'no endocervical cells seen' rate. If they do, the laboratory can make enquiries as to how they are taking their smears and suggest ways in which they can improve their technique.

Unfortunately, in this country, there is a good chance you simply won't know whether your smear showed endocervical cells or not, and there's really nothing you can do about it. However, if your smear report says 'No endocervical cells seen. Negative', should you have it repeated? I think the answer to this is yes, but not straight away. A repeat in a year seems sensible, just to be on the safe side. I do not think you should leave it 3 or 5 years before having a routine repeat smear.

Cervical ectopy or erosion

I was lying on the couch and the nurse was just asking me about my daughter, her son goes to the same school, when she suddenly said 'oh you've got an erosion'. I nearly stopped breathing.

This is another term that causes much unnecessary anxiety. It is a harmless appearance of the cervix, which is particularly common in young women, women who are pregnant, have had children, or who are taking the combined oral contraceptive pill. Those categories include a lot of people!

It just means that there are some soft, columnar cells on the outside surface of the cervix. Usually these cells stay inside the womb and the cervical canal. They have a good blood supply, so they appear red in colour. If they decide to move outwards, their red colour gives the surface of the cervix a 'grazed' look, which is why it was originally called an 'erosion'. Actually, nothing is being 'eroded' so the word is both inaccurate as well as rather frightening. For this reason we now call the appearance 'ectopy' or 'ectropion', derived from the Greek words meaning eversion, or turned inside out. It is quite harmless, but it can become a nuisance.

If an ectropion is large, you may notice more discharge than before. The discharge will be odourless and non-itchy, just like normal discharge. You may also notice some light bleeding after intercourse. All this is because the columnar cells are well supplied with blood vessels (causing bleeding) and glands (which produce discharge).

If the discharge or bleeding become a nuisance, it may be suggested that you can have the ectropion treated. This is most likely to be done by freezing the area, a procedure called cryotherapy ('kryos' means 'frost' in Greek). The treatment is done in an outpatient clinic and is very quick. A small, very cold metal instrument is pressed onto the cervix for a couple of minutes; you won't feel anything much at the time, though you may get some period-type pain. It is often a good idea to take a couple of painkillers beforehand just in case. Afterwards you are likely to have some discharge for several weeks, which is just the healing process. In fact, the discharge afterwards is by far the most tiresome part of the treatment and is the main reason for not treating an ectropion unless it is actually giving you problems. Sometimes the ectropion may gradually come back because the conditions which led to it are still there – another reason for not treating unless it is really bothersome.

Candida (thrush)

Candida is an extremely common infection, which happens to show up on a smear, but is not in any way related to cervical abnormalities. However, it can sometimes make the smear difficult to read and result in a borderline smear report – one of the good reasons for repeating those smears before doing anything else.

Candida, also popularly called thrush or yeast infection, is a fungus. It is a normal inhabitant of both the bowel and the vagina. Given half a chance it will multiply and occupy more and more space, resulting in a creamy, curd-like discharge. Indeed, this discharge led to its name, since 'candidus' means 'white' in Latin. The other thing you may notice is itching, often very intense, around the outside, the vulva. In many cases, however, candida simply shows up on testing either on an infection swab, or on a smear. Its other medical name, 'monilia' is derived from its bead-like appearance under the microscope ('monile' means 'necklace' in Latin).

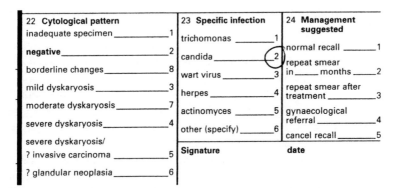

22 Cytological pattern	23 Specific infection	24 Management suggested
inadequate specimen ___1	trichomonas ___1	normal recall ___1
negative ___2	candida ___(2)	repeat smear in ___ months ___2
borderline changes ___8	wart virus ___3	
mild dyskaryosis ___3	herpes ___4	repeat smear after treatment ___3
moderate dyskaryosis ___7	actinomyces ___5	gynaecological referral ___4
severe dyskaryosis ___4	other (specify) ___6	
severe dyskaryosis/ ? invasive carcinoma ___5	Signature	cancel recall ___5
? glandular neoplasia ___6		date

Figure 3.3   Smear form showing candida.

The vagina is also normally inhabited by a number of bacteria. Not all bacteria are bad for you, some are positively helpful. One particularly good type is the lactobacillus, which produces lactic acid. As a result, the vagina is normally an acidic environment, which candida doesn't like very much. So it sits around, curled up in a corner, waiting for conditions to improve.

Anything that reduces the acidity of the vagina will help candida to grow. If you are given a course of antibiotics for an ear infection, those antibiotics will certainly kill off the nasty bacteria in your ear. Unfortunately, at the same time they will also wipe out nice lactobacillus. Candida suddenly wakes up: no acid! Antibiotics only work on bacteria, not fungi, so they will leave candida untouched and multiplying furiously.

If you are very run down, have the flu, or some other illness, your immune system will be busy fighting that and will have less time to think about candida. Again under those circumstances, attacks of thrush are more likely.

You can also reduce the acidity of your vagina by using perfumed bubble baths and soaps, as they are very alkaline. In some women, this will be enough to allow candida to multiply. Of course, if you are already suffering from an attack of thrush, you will make things very much worse if you then use such products. Biological washing powder will also make things worse, by attacking already sensitive skin.

Candida just loves the tropics. Heat and humidity are its favourite type of weather. In such conditions, or at any time if you are prone to thrush, you will find stockings better than tights and cotton underwear better than nylon.

Candida is very common in pregnancy, which is probably a combination of the immune system being somewhat depressed and the hormonal changes that occur. Nearly everyone thinks thrush is more common in women on the combined oral contraceptive pill, but scientific studies have not confirmed this. A great many women take the pill and a great many women get thrush; there is bound to be an overlap, which in the majority of cases is just coincidence.

Although candida is a normal inhabitant of the bowel, it may spread from there in large numbers into the vagina. This will help the vaginal thrush win its battle with lactobacillus (reinforcements!). Wiping backwards, not forwards, after a bowel motion will help prevent this happening. If the problem is recurrent and persistent, it is sometimes worth taking a course of anti-fungal tablets, usually nystatin, or, nowadays, Diflucan (fluconazole), to try and reduce the bowel candida population.

Vaginal thrush can make you feel as though you have cystitis, with irritation and burning when you pass urine. Unlike 'real' cystitis, bacteria will not be found in a urine sample sent for culture: the effect is local, at the entrance/exit of the urethra, rather than an actual bladder infection.

The treatment for thrush is usually a course of pessaries (which look like suppositories) and cream. The pessaries are put into the vagina at night, and the cream spread round the outside (the vulva) twice a day. Nowadays you can buy treatment over the counter at the chemist, in the form of Canesten, a strong pessary so only one is needed, and Canesten cream. It is often worth sharing a little of the cream with your partner; although candida is not a sexually transmitted disease, spores can travel backwards and forwards.

A newer treatment for thrush, which many women prefer, as it only involves swallowing one tablet, is Diflucan (fluconazole). This is just as effective as the pessaries and creams, without the mess (and is also available from the chemist). However, it is no better at preventing recurrences.

Some women (fortunately a small minority) have real problems with recurrent candida infection. It can make life very miserable if it keeps coming back literally every few weeks. In such cases, the most important thing is to scrupulously avoid all the things that make its life easier: the bubble baths, soaps, biological washing powder and so on.

Recurrent attacks are often prevented by using a pessary (such as Canesten 1) once a week regularly, whether or not you have symptoms, to try and keep the candida population down. Sometimes it is advised that you also use a pessary after having sex.

However, if you do have recurrent attacks of thrush, you would be best getting advice from a sexual health clinic (also called departments of genito-urinary medicine, or 'special' clinics). They have the most expertise at dealing with all vaginal infections, whether they are sexually transmitted or not. In addition, if the discharge is not going away with normal candida treatments, maybe it is not thrush at all, but something else. Many discharges are itchy, but may not be due to thrush at all. These clinics will do all the swab tests for you and will be able to give you at least part of the answer the same day.

Gardnerella

Gardnerella, also called 'anaerobic' or 'bacterial vaginosis', is another very common infection, this time by a bacterium. It should not be confused with the much more serious 'gonorrhoea' to which it is not in any way related.

21 CYTOLOGY REPORT

Clue cells suggestive of gardnerella

22 Cytological pattern	23 Specific infection	24 Management suggested
inadequate specimen _____1	trichomonas _____1	normal recall _____1
negative_____2	candida _____2	repeat smear in ____ months _____2
borderline changes_____8	wart virus _____3	
mild dyskaryosis_____3	herpes _____4	repeat smear after treatment _____3
moderate dyskaryosis_____7	actinomyces _____5	gynaecological referral_____4
severe dyskaryosis_____4	other (specify)_____(6)	cancel recall_____5
severe dyskaryosis/ ? invasive carcinoma _____5	**Signature**	**date**
? glandular neoplasia_____6		

Figure 3.4   Smear form result showing gardnerella.

Like candida, it is a normal inhabitant of the vagina and is usually not noticed at all. However, if it is present in large numbers, it can cause a discharge, which is not likely to be itchy but may smell slightly fishy, especially after intercourse.

'Clue cells' that may be mentioned on a smear report are normal cells to which the bacteria attach themselves. Together, they have a characteristic appearance under the microscope, giving a 'clue' that gardnerella may be present. They are not related to cervical abnormalities.

This condition is currently the subject of intense debate. Until recently, most doctors would only treat a woman if she actually complained of a smelly discharge, as it was thought to be quite harmless. However, there is now a suggestion that anaerobic vaginosis may play a part in pelvic inflammatory disease (PID or salpingitis), which can result in infertility. In addition, it has been linked with an increased risk of premature babies. It has not actually been proven to cause either of these problems, but doctors are now becoming interested in its possible role. Thus, the current tide of opinion is in favour of treatment with or without symptoms. But do you treat the partner for a condition which probably isn't sexually transmitted? Well, opinions are greatly divided on this: many clinics do not treat the partner. However, my view is that if you are going to treat a woman (particularly if it is a recurring problem), you might as well treat her partner in case it goes backwards and forwards between them, just like thrush. But it is very important that everyone concerned (and especially the couple) understand that it is just a precaution and no-one is laying blame at anyone's door. To have a row over something as uninteresting as gardnerella would really be a shame.

Two types of treatment are now available. The well-established method is a 5-day course of an antibiotic called metronidazole or Flagyl, 400 milligrams twice a day. It tastes disgusting (I believe Flagyl is the more palatable version) and you can't drink any alcohol while you are taking it: if you do, you will be quite unbelievably sick. The very unpleasantness of the treatment was one of the reasons why both doctors and their patients wondered if it was worthwhile.

A newer treatment is clindamycin (Dalacin) cream which is inserted into the vagina at night using an applicator. It should be used for 7 days. Although it may be a little messy, at least it has fewer side effects and appears to be as effective as metronidazole.

Of course, if you are being treated, you should not have sex until you have (both) finished the course, or you may just pass it back again.

Trichomonas

Trichomonas vaginalis is a one-celled organism, of a type known as a protozoan (in Greek, 'proto' means 'first' and 'zoion' means 'animal' – i.e. a very primitive animal). Trichomonas is fascinating to look at under the microscope, because it swims around, moving its hairs, or flagellae (so called because this is the Latin for 'whip', describing their whip-like motion).

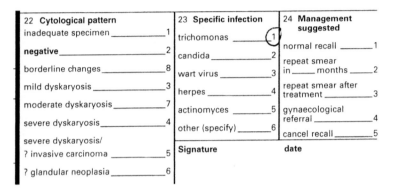

22 Cytological pattern	23 Specific infection	24 Management suggested
inadequate specimen ____1	trichomonas ____(1)	normal recall ____1
negative____2	candida ____2	repeat smear in ____ months ____2
borderline changes____8	wart virus ____3	repeat smear after treatment ____3
mild dyskaryosis ____3	herpes ____4	
moderate dyskaryosis____7	actinomyces ____5	gynaecological referral ____4
severe dyskaryosis____4	other (specify)____6	
severe dyskaryosis/ ? invasive carcinoma ____5	**Signature** date	cancel recall ____5
? glandular neoplasia____6		

Figure 3.5   Smear form result showing trichomonas.

As you can see from Figure 3.6, *Trichomonas vaginalis* is pear-shaped, with the flagellae at one end. It swims its way into your vagina during sex, though it is *just* possible to catch it from swimming pools or lavatory seats. Men usually have no symptoms and so do not realise they are passing it on. In fact, even tests for infection may not show it up in a man. However, although some women also have no symptoms, many get a nasty, frothy, itchy discharge, which smells of old fish. As with candida, the local irritation can make you feel as though you have cystitis.

Because of the intense inflammation it causes in the vagina and cervix, you can have bleeding after intercourse. The inflammation, and just the physical presence of these relatively large organisms, can also make it difficult to interpret a smear, so you may be asked to have a repeat smear after you have been treated. Although trichomonas can 'spoil' your smear, it does not cause abnormal cells to develop.

The treatment for trichomonas is actually the same as the traditional one for gardnerella, though they are not related. You – and definitely

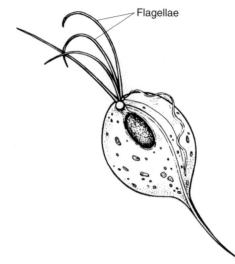

Flagellae

Figure 3.6   *Trichomonas vaginalis.*

also your partner – have to take a 5-day course of the antibiotic metronidazole (Flagyl), 400 milligrams twice a day (Dalacin cream has not been shown to be effective against trichomonas). Obviously, you must not have sex during this time, or you will reinfect each other. You also must not drink alcohol while taking metronidazole, or you will be very sick.

Unfortunately, trichomonas likes company. It is quite often the case that if you have been infected with it, you will find you have another infection as well. So it is always advisable to be tested at a genito-urinary medicine (sexual health) clinic, to be sure there is nothing else there.

Actinomyces-like organisms

Actinomyces is a bacterium which, once again, is a normal inhabitant of the bowel. However, in women who use an intrauterine contraceptive device (IUD), it very occasionally seems to migrate into the vagina. This seems to be more likely when the IUD is the older plastic, rather than copper-containing type. Because of its rarity and the fact that it cannot absolutely reliably be diagnosed on a smear, cytologists will usually say they have seen 'actinomyces-like organisms (ALOs)', rather than actual

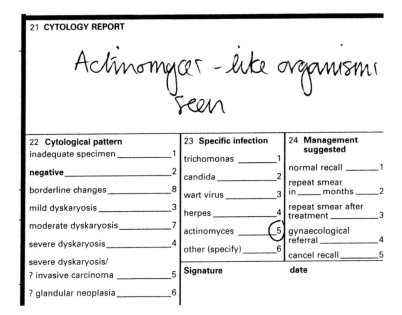

21 CYTOLOGY REPORT

Actinomyces - like organisms
seen

22 Cytological pattern	23 Specific infection	24 Management suggested
inadequate specimen _____1	trichomonas _____1	normal recall _____1
negative_____2	candida_____2	repeat smear
borderline changes_____8	wart virus_____3	in _____ months _____2
mild dyskaryosis _____3	herpes _____4	repeat smear after treatment _____3
moderate dyskaryosis_____7	actinomyces _____⑤	gynaecological
severe dyskaryosis_____4	other (specify)_____6	referral _____4
severe dyskaryosis/	**Signature**	cancel recall_____5
? invasive carcinoma _____5		**date**
? glandular neoplasia_____6		

Figure 3.7 Smear form showing that actinomyces-like organisms have been seen.

actinomyces (though this has been abbreviated on the report form to just 'actinomyces'). Actinomyces does not cause abnormal cells; once again it is being reported just for information.

Unfortunately, *very, very rarely* actinomyces can cause a potentially serious type of pelvic inflammatory disease (PID or salpingitis), which can lead to many problems, including infertility as a result of blocked Fallopian tubes. Thus, if your smear does show ALOs, your doctor will ask whether you have noticed any pain or discharge. You will be examined to make sure there are no signs that you need treatment. If not, you could just watch and wait, given that the number of cases of actual PID due to this organism is so small. You would have to be careful to seek advice if you had even the slightest twinge of pain or discharge. Many women cannot tolerate this kind of uncertainty and choose the other option, which is to have the current IUD removed and replaced immediately with another one. The new IUD should always be a copper-containing one.

Severe inflammatory changes – now properly called the borderline smear

I sincerely hope you will never see 'severe inflammatory changes' on a smear form. Indeed, I hope that I will never again see it on a smear report either. What does it mean? Don't ask me. In fact don't ask: nobody knows.

I'm not being funny. The category has actually been removed from the new smear form in an effort to try and stop cytologists using it. If used, it means completely different things to different people.

To some, inflammatory changes mean that there is an infection of some kind present, but they can't see anything specific (like candida or trichomonas). They can see a lot of white cells, which are pus cells, arriving to combat infection. However, to others, 'severe inflammation'

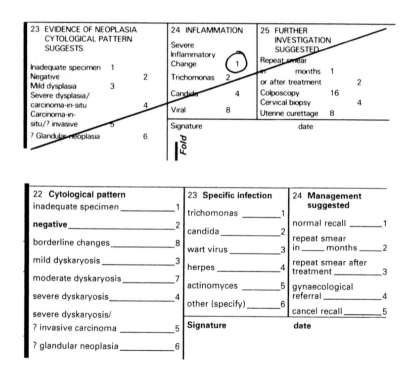

Figure 3.8 Old and new smear forms.

means the cells are showing minor changes, not enough to call it 'mild dyskaryosis' but not normal either – borderline abnormal cells, in fact. In this case, there may or may not be an infection present, but the important thing is that the cells are not quite normal. You will notice in Figure 3.8 that the new smear form has included a category called 'borderline changes' to force the cytologist to make a decision.

A smear reported properly as 'borderline change' is usually repeated after 6 months. If it is again abnormal, you are likely to have it repeated yet again, 6 months later. A third borderline smear means you will be referred for colposcopy. Studies have shown that in up to 30% of cases where there is a persistent borderline abnormality, there will be CIN present, of varying degrees of severity.

There is another reason why cells may look slightly abnormal. If you have gone past the menopause (change of life), your body stops producing the hormone oestrogen. This may make your vagina feel dry and the skin lining it (and everywhere else in your body) thin. These changes are called 'atrophic changes' from the Greek 'trophe', meaning 'nourishment' and the prefix 'a' which means 'without'. Cervical cells may also look 'atrophic', and then they can be difficult to distinguish from a borderline abnormality. In this case, it is often worth trying a short (6-week) course of vaginal oestrogen cream and then repeating the smear. If lack of oestrogen was the cause, the repeat smear is likely to be normal. If it is not, you should be referred for colposcopy.

4 HAVING A COLPOSCOPY EXAMINATION

I think the worst part was waiting an hour to be seen. I was getting more and more nervous all the time.

In some ways, it helped seeing other women who all had the same problem as myself. I started chatting to the person sitting next to me and found we live quite near each other. She wasn't so worried, as she'd had it all done before and was just coming back for a check-up. She made me feel a lot better.

Things have been improving in many colposcopy clinics, and the days of block booking everyone for the same time at the beginning of the clinic are over (I sincerely hope). Nevertheless, it is still likely you will have to wait to be seen. The chances are you will be anxious, even if you've been pretty level-headed so far. If possible, bring a friend or partner with you so that you have someone to talk to while you are waiting. That person may also be very useful when you are seeing the doctor: often you yourself are so nervous that afterwards you cannot remember much of what was said. Or you may find it difficult to ask questions, and your friend or partner can prompt you, or ask them for you.

You may be asked to change into a gown. Frankly, I have never seen the point of this. If you are wearing a loose skirt, all you need to do is take your panties and tights off once you are inside the examination room. Trousers and tight skirts are not a good idea as they definitely will have to come off, in which case you may want a gown to make yourself feel less exposed during the examination.

I wanted to ask so many questions. But when I was in with the doctor I couldn't think of them, I was nervous and muddled.

You may find it helpful to prepare a list of questions at home, in case they go out of your mind once you arrive. One thing you can definitely think about before you see the doctor is the date of your last period: I *guarantee* you will be asked. This is the single greatest time-wasting procedure I can think of. For the tenth time already that day, I ask 'when was your last period?' and suddenly there is a panic-stricken face in front of me. 'Oh, I think it was last month. I've got my diary here somewhere, just a minute. Erm . . . oh dear, I don't seem to have noted it down. No – here it is, the 27th.' Although it is sometimes nice to vegetate for a few minutes while this is going on, wouldn't you rather I, or whoever you are seeing, was using that time to answer some of your questions?

> I had a lot of things I wanted to ask. But there were so many people waiting, I felt I would be taking up too much time. The doctor was so busy.

Of course, if no-one opened their mouth except to say the date of their last period, clinics would be over in a fraction of the time. But although the doctors and nurses are busy, they are in fact there to look after you, and that includes answering your questions. Don't be put off; after all, how often do you get the opportunity to talk to an expert about what is wrong with you? Books, leaflets, friends and the internet are all very well for general information and advice, but you will only be able to find out what specifically applies to you from the doctor doing the examination.

The doctor may also ask you some questions relating to your periods, your method of contraception, whether or not you smoke and your general medical history. This does not usually take very long; most of the discussion will be about your smear and what it all means. Bear in mind that some of the answers to your questions can only be given after the examination has taken place and the doctor has had a look at the area of abnormality.

The examination

Lurking in the background, you will notice a funny-looking couch, angled slightly and with the bottom end missing. Instead it will have leg rests or stirrups. You will be asked to lie down on it so that your bottom is right at the end of the couch. Depending on the type of couch, your knees will be lying on top of knee rests, or in stirrups, or they will be bent and your feet positioned in foot rests. No matter how it is done it is very inelegant, but this position makes it easier to see your cervix. (The womb is actually quite mobile and will change its angle according to your

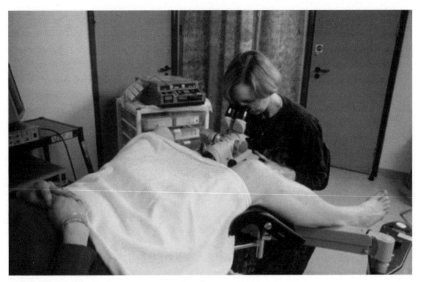

Figure 4.1   The colposcopy examination.

position.) Indeed, in many other countries, women usually also have their smears taken lying on this type of couch. I am always having to stop bewildered American women in particular shuffling down to the end of our conventional clinic couches, trying to find the stirrups!

It was really good having the nurse there. She was very friendly and chatted to me, even held my hand while I was having the biopsy. Actually, it wasn't so bad, but it made me feel better, that she was there.

Some clinics now have video equipment so that you can actually watch your own examination taking place. Not everyone likes this, so don't feel intimidated, you can always ask to have it switched off. Sometimes there are pictures on the ceiling or on an adjacent wall to keep your mind occupied. There may even be soft music! I have seen women bring a personal stereo along: then you can listen to music of your own choice. All clinics have nurses who will do their best to put you at your ease and make you feel comfortable.

It was horrible. Suddenly, there was a crowd of people standing at the end of the couch, all looking at me. I think they were students. The doctor seemed more interested in talking to them than to me.

49

Unfortunately, colposcopy has to be taught to other doctors, and the only way to learn is by practical training. However, you should never have to put up with the sort of experience described above. For a start, you have the right to refuse any other doctor or student being in the room. Indeed, the doctor should first ask for your permission to have another person there, not just herd strangers in. And it is very intimidating to have several other people there: one extra is enough.

I have also seen clinics where doctors and students walk in and out of rooms while women are being examined. There you are, nether regions exposed, while strange men suddenly appear. They may know they are doctors, but as far as you are concerned they could be Joe Bloggs. Hopefully, this type of behaviour is on the way out, but one way of preventing it is to ask for the door to be locked while you are being examined.

Anyway, hopefully you are lying comfortably on a couch, perhaps listening to soothing music and gazing at an interesting picture. There will now be some fumbling around while the doctor gets the colposcope into position. Although it is quite a large, intimidating instrument, all it really comprises is a magnifying glass and a light source. The light illuminates your cervix and the magnifying glass enables the doctor to see what is going on. It is that simple.

No part of the colposcope enters you. Instead, a speculum (hopefully warmed) is inserted into your vagina, just as for a smear. However, this speculum will stay in longer than for a smear, usually about 5 minutes. Again, as with smears, the more you can relax the less uncomfortable the procedure will be.

Your cervix will then be wiped with some cotton wool soaked in dilute acetic acid. Acetic acid is the technical term for vinegar, and indeed, you may detect the familiar smell in the room. The acetic acid may sting a little and feel cold, but it doesn't hurt. For reasons we do not yet fully understand, acetic acid stains abnormal areas white, and the degree of whiteness is one of the features that help the doctor decide the degree of abnormality. It takes a little time for the white areas to show up, so at this point you will probably find yourself discussing the weather, your job, where you are going on holiday . . . .

Sometimes the doctor will then also put some iodine on your cervix, again using a cotton swab. This is another way of showing up abnormal areas: they do not go dark brown as you would expect; instead they stay pale yellow. Because the contrast between dark brown/pale yellow is greater than that between white/pink, iodine is a good way of 'double-checking' that no abnormal area has been missed. It also makes it easier to see the size of the area. If iodine is used, you will get a dark brown discharge for a couple of days.

If there is an abnormal-looking area on your cervix, the doctor will take a tiny piece from it called a biopsy. The biopsy is about the size of a pin-head and you could liken the procedure to having a cut on your finger. Many women are actually unaware anything has happened, others feel a short, sharp pain. However, most women do have a mild period pain afterwards and some feel a little sick, as you can when you are having period pain. In order to prevent this, it may be helpful to take a painkiller beforehand – preferably about 15–20 minutes in advance, to give it time to work. There is a painkiller designed for period pain, called Ponstan, or mefenamic acid, which is often good in this situation; unfortunately it is only available on prescription. A more easily available alternative is Nurofen or ibuprofen, which you can buy over the counter at the chemist. It will not make you drowsy, but is related to aspirin, so it is best taken with some food, or it can upset your stomach.

You are likely to have some bleeding after a biopsy, just as you would if you cut your finger, so a tampon is often put in for you before the speculum is removed. Alternatively, a special solution called Monsel's, or silver nitrate sticks may be used to stop the bleeding. At last the whole thing is over; you will probably be surprised to find how quick it really was. You are likely to have some bleeding for a couple of days afterwards. It's a good idea to make sure you have the phone number of the clinic in case you have any queries or get worried.

A word about 'acetowhite change'

Much of the technique of colposcopy is based on the white appearance that occurs when dilute acetic acid is wiped across the cervix. This phenomenon was first described in the 1930s and the procedure adopted with enthusiasm – but without understanding why it actually happens. At first, doctors thought that everything that became white was abnormal, but it is now known that this is not the case. Although abnormal areas do turn white, the same thing will happen in a number of normal conditions. For example, areas of cells undergoing the normal process of squamous metaplasia (see Chapter 2) will turn white. In fact, cells involved in any kind of change, normal or abnormal, seem to go white.

It is important that you understand a very important and very simple concept: not everything that turns white with acetic acid is abnormal. This means that 'false alarms' occur. I sometimes see women who are actually worried when I tell them the good news that their biopsy showed no abnormal cells. 'But didn't you say you saw something that might be abnormal?' Well, now you can understand why that may be wrong.

After the examination

The biopsy specimen is placed in a preservative solution (formalin) and sent away to a laboratory. There it will be studied very carefully under a microscope. The biopsy gives a more accurate result than a smear, which is not really surprising: after all, a smear is just some loose cells, while a biopsy is a small, but solid piece of tissue. Although abnormal cells look different individually, they are also arranged in different ways: in a mild abnormality, CIN 1, only one-third of the cells above the basement membrane are abnormal. In CIN 2, two-thirds of the cells are abnormal, while in CIN 3 all the cells are abnormal (see Figure 4.2).

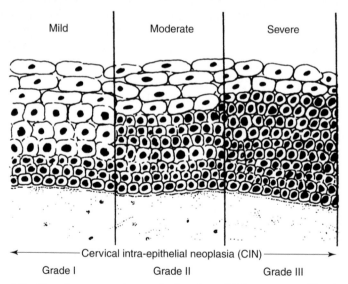

Figure 4.2 The changes on the cervical surface (CIN), as reported by the pathologist from the biopsies.

Obviously, you cannot see the extent of the abnormal cells if they are loose; you need a solid area, which is exactly what is provided by a biopsy.

The results of the biopsy usually take a week or two to come back. So although the doctor who has examined you will be able to give you his or her impression of the degree of abnormality, you will not get a definite answer on the same day. This is a shame, as waiting always involves anxiety, but there is no alternative. Usually, at least the doctor will have been able to reassure you that you do not have cancer, which for many women is the most important thing. It is more difficult to predict grades of CIN accurately; in addition, as mentioned above, not everything that stains up white will actually turn out to be CIN. So you may find there is nothing wrong after all.

You may be made another appointment to come back for your biopsy result. Alternatively, you may be notified by post or sometimes by telephone. The actual procedure will depend on individual doctors and clinics.

Once the biopsy result is known, the next step is to decide what type of treatment, if any, will be best. You may not need any treatment, and will just be asked to come back for another colposcopy examination at a later date. If you do need treatment, there are several different kinds, which we shall be looking at in Chapter 5. The type used in your particular case will depend on several factors:

- the degree of abnormality
- the preference of the doctor
- what is actually available at the clinic.

'See and treat' clinics

In recent years, some clinics have been offering the option of being treated on the same day as your initial colposcopy. The advantage is that you are spared an extra visit to the clinic; normally you would have a colposcopy and then would come back another time for treatment, if the biopsy result confirmed that you needed it. This saves you time and obviously saves the clinic money, since they only have to book you in once, not twice.

Some women prefer this. If you are busy, taking time to come to the clinic can be a nuisance. Also, if you are treated straight away, you do not have to go on thinking about what might be wrong with you – it has already been removed.

I think 'see and treat' clinics are quite reasonable for women who have a smear result showing moderate or severe dyskaryosis. Because smears get more accurate at higher grades of abnormality, there is a good chance that you will in fact have CIN 2 or 3 and therefore would need treatment. In that case, it can well be a good option to have it done straight away, as long as you are prepared for that to happen.

There are two main disadvantages. The first is a medical one: you may be treated unnecessarily, because the result of the biopsy will not yet be known. So the doctor may think you have CIN 2, but the biopsy turns out to show only borderline changes, or may even be normal. In an ordinary clinic, the result of the biopsy would have indicated that you did not need treatment, but meanwhile, in a 'see and treat' clinic, the treatment will already have been done.

The second disadvantage, in my view, is that it can be too sudden. There you are, incredibly nervous, only taking in half of what is being said to you. You are only just beginning to understand what may be wrong – and you've been treated. Now some women may actually prefer this, as they don't have time to get panic-stricken about the treatment. But others may feel totally out of control. You have no time to go away and think about it, discuss it. You might have preferred the option of being monitored for a while to see if you get better without treatment – a not unreasonable thing to do if you have CIN 1.

As we will see in the next chapter, most treatments nowadays are very quick and simple, so it is not the actual treatment that is a problem. But afterwards, your activities will be restricted, so you may need to plan for this in advance (this is discussed in detail in Chapter 5). You may have planned a holiday in the next couple of weeks, it might be your anniversary, your partner has planned a surprise romantic weekend – and now suddenly you can't have intercourse. So, if you are going to a 'see and treat' clinic, you should in fact assume you are going to be treated and make all the arrangements, knowing they may have to be cancelled if you are not treated. And all this before you even know what is wrong with you!

'See and treat' clinics are very attractive to administrators because they save money, and they can save time for both doctors and women. But do not feel pressurised. You still have the option of saying you would rather wait for the biopsy result and come back, if you prefer.

Unsatisfactory colposcopy

Occasionally, a colposcopy examination may be considered technically unsatisfactory. This happens when the doctor sees an abnormal-looking area which stretches backwards into the cervical canal, but he or she cannot see where it ends. Although what is visible may look mild, how can you be sure that the 'invisible' part isn't worse? So then the only way of finding out is to actually remove the abnormal area with a cone biopsy, described in the Chapter 5.

In this situation you will probably not have a conventional biopsy first; you will be made a separate appointment to come back for the treatment. The cone biopsy then provides both the piece of tissue that can be studied in the laboratory and the treatment at the same time.

A colposcopy may occasionally also be unsatisfactory even if the doctor does not see anything that looks abnormal. A situation may occur where you have been referred with an abnormal smear, but the doctor cannot see the whole of the transformation zone (the area in which abnormal cells are most likely to occur). Everything he can see is normal, but again an abnormality in the 'invisible' area cannot be ruled out.

Having an unsatisfactory colposcopy does not mean anything sinister. It does not mean you are more likely to have cancer. It just means

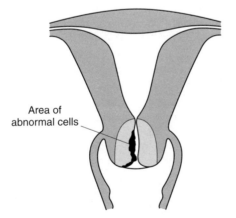

Area of abnormal cells

Figure 4.3 Abnormal-looking area extending high into the cervical canal.

the position of your abnormal area (or your transformation zone) made it impossible to get a complete view at colposcopy. It is worth mentioning that the chances of this actually happening to you are very small: the vast majority of colposcopies are technically perfectly satisfactory.

5 TREATMENT OPTIONS FOR CIN

The last 20 years have seen great progress in the methods of treatment available for cervical abnormalities. The advent of colposcopy allowed the abnormal area to be properly assessed before treatment, but this would have been of limited use if the treatment options had not also improved.

This chapter covers ways of treating cervical intra-epithelial neoplasia (CIN); the treatment of cancer will be discussed in Chapter 6. There are now five treatment options available:

- cryotherapy
- electrocautery
- cold coagulation
- laser treatment (which can either be a vaporisation or an excision)
- loop diathermy.

All of them aim to remove the abnormal cells, either by destroying them, or by cutting them out, while causing as little damage as possible to the surrounding normal tissues. To an extent, the choice you are offered will depend on the preferences of your gynaecologist and on what is actually available at the hospital. Since laser and loop diathermy are now the treatments most in favour, I shall describe them first.

Laser vaporisation and loop diathermy

I shall discuss these two treatments together, since, although they are technically different, from your point of view they are very similar. They are both usually done under local anaesthetic, take only a few minutes, require the same aftercare and have the same low frequency of long-term complications. But first I shall explain the principles behind them.

57

Laser vaporisation

The word laser is derived from 'light amplification by stimulated emission of radiation'. The basic principle is that the machine produces a very fine, and therefore very concentrated and powerful, beam of light. Ordinary light 'sprays out', so its energy is lessened by being spread around more thinly. A laser machine manages to concentrate the light rays so that they stay in line; thus, the energy is harnessed more effectively (see Figure 5.1)

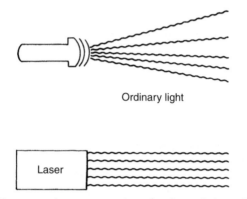

Ordinary light

Laser

Figure 5.1 Diagrammatic representation of ordinary light and laser light.

This beam can then be moved around by means of mirrors and lenses. In addition, the amount of energy it contains can be varied by changing the width of the beam: the narrower the beam, the more concentrated the energy.

As you know, light produces heat: think how hot a light bulb is if you touch it. The heat in a laser beam is so intense that it causes cells to literally evaporate into thin air. This is why the process is called 'laser vaporisation'.

If the beam is made very fine, it will cut through cells like a knife; the laser can therefore also be used to remove pieces of tissue, as for a cone biopsy, which is discussed later.

A laser machine needs to be attached physically to a colposcope, because it relies on the lens in the colposcope itself. This is a disadvantage, because only the more expensive types of colposcope can be attached to a laser. When you think that a laser machine itself costs around £30 000, if you then also have to use a colposcope costing over

£10 000, the expense is considerable. (Ordinary colposcopes cost around £5000.)

A laser machine looks like a large box, with a steel tube coming out for attachment to the colposcope. The light beam is conducted down the arm to the colposcope and is then directed on to the cervix using the lenses and mirrors in the colposcope. Although the beam itself is invisible, it is accompanied by a red light so that it can be seen. Because of the potential problem of the beam being reflected back into the faces of the doctor and nurse, they are likely to wear protective glasses. Indeed, although you are much less at risk, in some units you may also be offered glasses.

By looking through the colposcope, the beam can be guided with great precision to ensure that only the abnormal tissue is removed, with very little damage to the normal areas.

Loop diathermy

The correct name for this is actually 'large loop excision of the transformation zone', shortened to LLETZ (or LEEP in the USA). Although the basic idea of using hot wire loops to excise areas of the cervix is not new, its introduction as a form of treatment dates only from around 1987. However, it has rapidly taken over from the laser as the most popular method of treatment.

The basic principle is that a thin wire is heated electrically to a high temperature and cuts through the cervical tissue rather like a cheese wire cuts through cheese. Because the wire is very thin and can be guided exactly by looking through the colposcope, the area excised is accurate and the damage to adjacent normal tissue is minimal, as with the laser.

One advantage of the loop method is that it is much cheaper than the laser. The machine that supplies the electrical energy is relatively cheap, at between £3000 and £6000. In addition, it does not need to be directly connected to a colposcope, so a cheaper type is quite adequate. This has meant that the technique is not restricted to large, well-funded units, and brings the benefits previously associated with the laser to a wider public.

There is another advantage of the loop which has, in many experts' eyes, placed it ahead of laser vaporisation. Whereas the laser evaporates the cells away, never to be seen again, the loop preserves them, allowing the piece of cervix removed to be sent for examination in the pathology laboratory. This means that the whole abnormal area can be checked, not

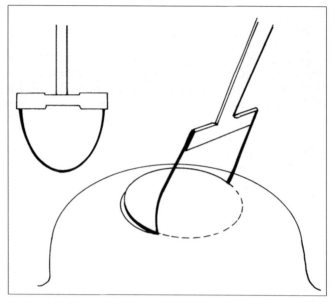

Figure 5.2   Loop diathermy in use.

just the tiny area taken in a punch biopsy (see Chapter 4). Use of the loop has shown that punch biopsies are not always representative of the whole area: for example, a punch biopsy may show CIN 2 (the second stage of abnormal cells), but the loop specimen removed at treatment shows there is also some CIN 3. Occasionally, previously unsuspected early cancers have been found by examining the loop specimen; these had not been diagnosed by the doctor doing the colposcopy, and were not evident from the punch biopsy. If a laser vaporisation had been performed, no-one would ever have known – until the woman developed problems if the cancer had not been completely removed by the treatment. This is another advantage of loop diathermy: when the piece of cervix is examined in the laboratory, they can tell if the whole abnormal area has been removed, because if it has, the edges of the piece will be free of abnormality. This is important information, especially for CIN 3, since, if some has been left behind, the doctor is alerted to arrange particularly careful follow-up. It does not, however, usually mean you need another treatment straight away, as the abnormal cells left behind may yet be dealt with by your own immune system.

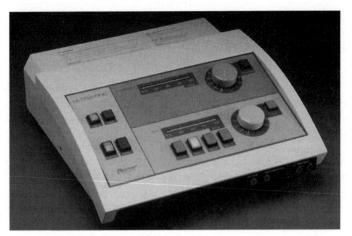

Figure 5.3 A loop diathermy machine.

Although the loop has all these advantages, laser is still a perfectly viable option. The laser can also be used to remove pieces of tissue, by making the beam very fine, although this does take longer and is a little more difficult than with the loop. Small treatments performed in this way are called laser excisions, as opposed to cone biopsies, which are larger (see below). If a doctor has become very good at using the laser for excision, the chances are you will not notice much difference. And some doctors are worried that the loop is too easy: it is tempting to overtreat, simply because it is such a simple procedure. Nevertheless, at present, the majority of experts are in favour of loop diathermy.

What happens during a laser or loop diathermy treatment

Both procedures are usually done in the outpatient clinic under local anaesthetic, unless there is some special reason why a general anaesthetic is necessary. This is sometimes the case if the area to be treated is very large, or for some reason it is difficult for the doctor to have a good view of the cervix.

Most doctors prefer not to perform the treatment during the heavy days of a period, although light bleeding is not a problem. Heavy bleeding can obscure the view, making the procedure more difficult, and also you are then more likely to have heavy bleeding during and after the treatment, because the cervix is already 'in the mood' for bleeding. If you are due a period when you are booked for treatment, it is worth phoning the clinic to check whether you should come.

Having booked the childminder and got my mother organised to stay for the weekend, I suddenly realised I was going to have my period just at the time of the treatment. Typical. But, when I rang, the doctor said as I was on the pill, I could just run two packets together to avoid having a bleed that month. She said it was quite safe to do that.

Postponing a bleed is very easy if you are on the pill. The only exception is if you are taking a triphasic type of pill, which has three different doses and will have three different colours of pills. In this case, you would need to keep taking the last row of pills from other packets in order to maintain the same dose level.

Try and bring someone with you. Although both types of treatment only take a few minutes, many women feel a little 'shaky' afterwards, often because they have been so anxious. It is nice then to have someone there, even better if they have a car in which to take you home.

You may be given some painkillers when you go in. These are usually Ponstan (mefenamic acid), designed to stop you having period-type cramps after the treatment. They are similar to Nurofen (ibuprofen) and are given at the start in order that they should have time to work.

Since the first part of the procedure involves a colposcopy, the same principles apply: again, a loose skirt is a good idea, since you will not need to take it off. You will sit on the same type of couch as for a colposcopy, with your legs resting on rests or in stirrups. The doctor will then do a colposcopy (see Chapter 4) in order to locate the abnormal area. Then he or she will put in the local anaesthetic. This is done in much the same way as at the dentist (except, of course, it is your cervix, not your gum, which is being injected!) and indeed, many clinics actually use dental syringes and needles. Unfortunately, just as at the dentist, this can be the worst part of the procedure. Not everyone feels the injection, but some women do find it unpleasant. However, it is over quite quickly and then you should be numb for the treatment itself.

The local anaesthetic needs a few minutes to work, which is why you will find yourself discussing the weather, your job, the latest film releases and so on. When the doctor is ready to start the treatment, you will hear a hissing noise, which is a suction machine being switched on. This is attached by tubing to the speculum (the metal instrument in your vagina) and simply removes any unpleasant odour caused by the treatment. The treatment itself can also make a little noise: you may notice a beeping sound.

If you are being treated by loop diathermy, a special pad will be stuck onto your thigh in order to 'earth' you: unfortunately, this also provides a free leg waxing treatment when it is removed.

I was surprised at how quick the actual treatment was. Most of the time was spent talking beforehand and waiting for the anaesthetic to work. Once he started, I could hear a noise and I felt a bit hot inside once or twice, but it was over so fast. I didn't feel any pain and it can't have taken more than a couple of minutes.

Afterwards, you may be asked to lie down for a few minutes in another room, just to calm down and make sure there is no bleeding. It is at this time that some women feel a little faint – and we don't want you to keel over in the corridor! You may be given some antiseptic cream to put into your vagina at night. However, there is no evidence this really does protect against infection, so many doctors have now stopped advising its use. Remember to bring a sanitary towel with you, as not all clinics have them – and if they do, they may be non-adhesive and resemble nappies. Tampons are not suitable, as discussed below.

After the treatment

You will need to go home and rest for the remainder of the day. You will probably feel remarkably well, which is the biggest problem. Your cervix needs time to heal: there is a raw wound on which a clot is trying to form. Gravity is against it because whenever you stand up, your cervix is pointing downwards, so the clot may drop off. And if you do any heavy lifting, running, jumping, aerobics, horse riding, housework (yes, you finally have a medical excuse), it has no chance. Basically, you need to become a couch potato for a while. This is the time to watch all those videos, read lots of books and take up knitting.

Exercise of a different kind is also bad news: the last thing your cervix needs right now is to be hit. So no penetrative sexual intercourse for 4 weeks after the treatment and, for the 4 weeks after that, only with a condom. Remember raw wounds are prone to infection. For the same reason, no tampons and no swimming for the first 4 weeks. You will need to invest in 'Super Plus' sanitary towels (such a joy).

It is quite normal, unfortunately, to bleed for up to 4 weeks after the treatment. The bleeding can take many forms: a watery discharge, spotting, or even resemble a period. It can stop for days, weeks even, and then start again at random. You are much more likely to bleed if you ignore the advice about taking it easy: the temptation is enormous because you will be feeling really well.

It is not advisable to go on long journeys, or to travel to exotic countries within the first 4 weeks: although you might think this is good time to go away, what will you do on a beach in the middle of nowhere if you suddenly start to bleed heavily and are worried?

If you do have heavy bleeding, the first thing to do is to put yourself to bed and take some painkillers if you are getting cramps. Ponstan (mefenamic acid) or Nurofen (ibuprofen) are likely to be best, but paracetamol should also be adequate. In most cases, the bleeding will diminish if you just rest. If you are very worried, call the hospital or clinic where you were treated; they will give you advice and may arrange to see you, occasionally even to admit you overnight. Obviously, if you are too far away, call your GP or go to the local hospital Accident and Emergency department. If you go into hospital, the chances are you will simply lie in a bed there instead of at home. However, very occasionally the bleeding really is enough of a problem to warrant medical treatment, a stitch or cautery using the laser or the diathermy machine.

Although all these instructions and warnings may seem rather frightening, the vast majority of women have no problems at all and wonder what all the fuss was about. But, to say it again, don't be tempted to overdo it because you feel so well.

If you have an intrauterine contraceptive device (IUD)

I was stunned when the doctor said 'Oh, you've got a coil, that'll have to come out' and just whipped it out there and then. No-one had said anything to me beforehand.

Unfortunately, IUDs may (though not always) need to be removed before the treatment as the threads can get cut off, making subsequent removal much more difficult. However, you do not want to be taken by surprise because you might become pregnant. IUDs work in retrospect, so if you have had otherwise unprotected sex in the week prior to removal, you could still become pregnant. The best thing to do is either to arrange an alternative method of contraception well before the treatment, or to use an additional method, such as the condom, for the week before.

Follow-up

Most clinics will arrange to see you for a colposcopy and smear between 4 and 9 months after the treatment. If a smear is taken sooner than 4 (some doctors would now even say 6) months after treatment, it seems more likely to give a falsely abnormal result – this is because cells that are regenerating can be difficult to distinguish from cells that are abnormal.

Often one follow-up colposcopy is usually all you need. If everything is fine, you will then simply have yearly smears. However, if you were treated for CIN 3, or there is any worry that some abnormal cells may have been left behind, it is likely you will be seen at least once more for colposcopy, just to be on the safe side. The timing and frequency of follow-up visits varies greatly from clinic to clinic, depending on an individual doctor's preference and the resources available.

What is the chance of the treatment failing?

There is a 90–95% chance that you will only require one treatment, so the success rate is very good indeed. In general, the larger the area requiring treatment and the greater the degree of abnormality, the higher the chance that a second treatment will be required.

Are there any long-term problems?

My friend had to have treatment some years ago and then she had two miscarriages one after the other when she tried for a baby. It took them 3 years before they managed to have Joe.

When the only method of treatment was surgical, using a scalpel (knife), there was a risk of problems. A larger amount of tissue was removed than was really necessary, resulting in difficulties becoming pregnant and also in a higher risk of miscarriage and premature babies. One of the great advantages of both these newer treatments is that there is very little risk of any of these problems.

Other forms of treatment

There are three other types of treatment, cryotherapy, cold coagulation and electrocautery. These are less used nowadays because laser and loop diathermy are more versatile and have become more popular. However, they are perfectly valid methods in certain circumstances.

The post-treatment instructions for all three methods are the same, and are similar to those following laser or loop diathermy, so, to avoid repetition, I shall give them here. Following all these treatments you are likely to have a watery, blood-stained discharge or frank bleeding for between 4 and 6 weeks. You will be asked to avoid penetrative sexual intercourse and the use of tampons for about the same length of time. It is also a good idea to avoid strenuous exercise for at least 3 weeks.

Cryotherapy

The word 'kryos' means 'frost' in Greek, and indeed, this method works by freezing the cells. The instrument used is called a cryoprobe and is

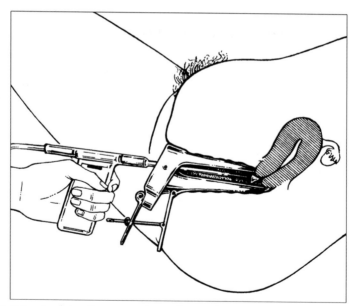

Figure 5.4   Applying the cryoprobe to the cervix.

attached to a pressurised supply of carbon dioxide or nitrous oxide gas. When the pressure is suddenly released, the gas shoots down the inside of the metal rod up to the tip, making it very cold. (In fact, its temperature goes down to around –60°C.) The tip of the cryoprobe is pressed onto the cervix and held there for about 3 minutes. One application (of only 1 or 2 minutes) is enough to treat a cervical ectopy (see Chapter 3), but if CIN is being treated, the probe is then removed for about 5 minutes before being reapplied for another 3-minute dose.

Cryotherapy is a simple treatment, for which a local anaesthetic is not needed. However, you would be well advised to have some painkillers beforehand, as you are likely to feel a dull ache, or period-type cramps.

Because it is difficult to guarantee the depth – and the width – of treatment using cryotherapy, its use is limited to small areas of abnormality whose severity does not exceed CIN 2 (the second stage of abnormal cells). It is also used for the treatment of cervical ectopy. However, it can cause some scarring of the cervix, which may make follow-up more difficult. Its main advantages are that it is cheap, easy to do and does not require any anaesthetic.

Electrodiathermy

This should not be confused with loop diathermy, with which it has little in common. The principle is not too dissimilar from cryotherapy: an electrode is applied to the cervix, but this time heat is used, at 1000°C.

Electrodiathermy has to be performed under general anaesthetic, because it would be very painful. The electrode is held on until no more mucus is seen coming from the cervical glands. In this way, the depth of treatment is known to be adequate, even for areas of CIN 3: abnormal cells are very unlikely to extend below the level of the glands.

Although electrodiathermy is an effective treatment for all degrees of CIN, the fact that it has to be performed under a general anaesthetic makes it unattractive nowadays, especially in comparison with laser and loop diathermy treatments.

Cold coagulation

Although its name suggests a cold temperature, in fact this method uses heat. It is only 'cold' by comparison with electrodiathermy. This time a small probe is heated to 100°C. It is applied to the cervix for 20-second intervals and the whole treatment only lasts a minute or two.

Cold coagulation does not require an anaesthetic and leaves no scarring. You may feel some dull, period-type pain during the treatment, so it is a good idea to take a couple of painkillers beforehand. This technique can be used for all grades of CIN.

If you need a general anaesthetic

Nowadays very few women need to have a general anaesthetic for treatment of cervical abnormalities. However, as mentioned earlier, if the area requiring treatment is particularly large or inaccessible, or if you are very nervous, a general anaesthetic may be advised. A general anaesthetic is also more likely to be advised if you need a cone biopsy (see below).

Many hospitals will now admit you as a 'day case', so you come in early, having not eaten or drunk anything since midnight. You will be seen by a junior doctor or a nurse practitioner who will ask some questions and examine your chest, to make sure there is no danger in having the anaesthetic. If you have a chest infection or even just a cold it is unlikely they will go ahead and you will have to return another day.

> The worst thing was the hanging around, waiting for things to happen. I was nervous and just couldn't concentrate on the book I'd brought. If I had to do it again I'd bring something really light, some magazines or a detective story or something. The woman in the next bed had just had her operation and was fast asleep, so I couldn't talk to her, but I had a chat with someone else who'd had my operation done 2 days ago. She seemed OK, which made me feel a bit better.

Just before you are taken into the operating theatre, you will be given a sedative injection or tablet. The next thing you know you will be waking up feeling groggy and perhaps a little sore. It is very important someone comes to collect you if you are going home the same day as you are unlikely to be fully 'with it' for several hours at least. And again, remember the sanitary towels.

If you have to stay in overnight, the procedure is much the same, but is even more tedious since you are there longer. Most people find it hard to sleep in hospital wards; there is always noise, people walking around, telephones ringing. You may be offered a sleeping tablet, it is up to you whether you want to take it. If you are having a cone biopsy, you may

68

have to stay in for a couple of days afterwards as well. Although you may think beforehand that you don't want visitors, I would advise you to have some, as you will be crawling up the wall with boredom before too long.

An abnormal smear in pregnancy

This can be a problem because treatment is best avoided if at all possible. Even after a biopsy, bleeding can be a problem. Fortunately, the vast majority of abnormalities can safely be left for 9 months, until the baby has been safely delivered. Remember that the cells take a long time to develop through all the stages of abnormality to actual cancer.

However, you will be monitored during the pregnancy and are likely to have at least one colposcopy (though biopsies are also usually avoided because of problems with bleeding) to check the area. In the vast majority of cases there are no problems.

What happens if you are found to have early cancer while you are pregnant? This is always a difficult problem. There are many factors to be considered, including the degree of cancer and how far the pregnancy has progressed. Does the hospital, or one nearby, have good facilities for looking after premature babies? Each individual case is different.

> I just don't know what to do. I'm only 8 weeks and the doctor says the safest thing would be for me to have a termination. But they want me to have a hysterectomy so this is my only chance of ever having a baby. Jim and I have wanted children so much, it would make us so happy to have just one. But what if the cancer spreads before I have the operation?

You will need to talk through all the options with your gynaecologist. Ultimately, it is you and your partner who have to live with the consequences of any decision you reach, so you need to have thought about it very carefully.

Cone biopsy

As its name suggests, a cone biopsy removes a cone-shaped piece of the cervix (see Figure 5.5). Before the introduction of colposcopy, this was the standard treatment for an abnormal smear; however, because in those days it involved a general anaesthetic and had long-term complications, only women whose smears persistently showed severe

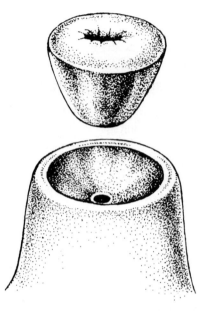

Figure 5.5 Cone biopsy.

dyskaryosis were treated. Nowadays, it is only performed under three circumstances:

- if the abnormal area extends so far up into the cervical canal that its upper limit cannot be seen through the colposcope. The doctor may be quite happy that he/she cannot see any evidence of cancer, but what about the abnormal area which is not visible? There is always the danger that something will be missed.
- if a woman's smear keeps showing severe dyskaryosis but no abnormality can be seen on colposcopy to account for that result. Usually, if this happens, the doctor will repeat the smear first to make sure it was not a mistake. If it again shows severe dyskaryosis, a cone biopsy will be advised.
- if, on colposcopy, the doctor is worried that the abnormal area may be starting to turn into an early cancer. In this case, the cone biopsy performs a dual function: by removing a relatively large piece of the cervix, hopefully it will remove all the abnormal area. In addition, as discussed in the section on loop diathermy, the piece of

tissue will be looked at very carefully in the laboratory to see exactly what was there, and whether the edges are clear of abnormality. In this way, the cone biopsy provides a diagnosis and at the same time, the treatment.

The term 'cone biopsy' is really rather misleading as it is often confused with the tiny punch biopsy taken during colposcopy. Whereas a punch biopsy just gives information about what abnormality is present, a cone biopsy also, in most cases, will remove the abnormality as well. Thus, cone biopsy is really a form of treatment, which is why it is included in this chapter.

Whereas the majority of women having a colposcopy will have a tiny punch biopsy taken, only around 10% cent will need a cone biopsy.

There are now three possible ways of performing a cone biopsy: surgically ('knife cone biopsy') or by using the laser or large loop diathermy.

Surgical ('knife') cone biopsy

If you are to have a surgical cone biopsy, you will need to stay in hospital for a couple of days. If you are due your period on the date booked, the surgeon may prefer to reschedule the operation, so it is worth ringing up to check.

The operation is short, lasting only about 20 minutes, but you will need to have a light general anaesthetic (see the section above). Usually, you come into hospital the day before the operation and stay for a day or two afterwards. You are likely to have some period-type pain for a day or two and also to bleed for several days. Indeed, you may bleed on and off for several weeks after the operation. The post-treatment advice is the same as for laser or loop diathermy treatment (see earlier sections).

Surgical cone biopsy can result in several problems. First, the external cervical os (entrance to the cervical canal) can become very tight afterwards. The technical term for this is 'stenosis' from the Greek word 'stenos', meaning narrow. If this happens, your periods may be painful and it may be very difficult to obtain an adequate cervical smear. By contrast, the internal cervical os may become too slack. This may occur if the cone biopsy had to be made long, because the area of abnormality was high up in the cervical canal (see Figure 5.6).

If the muscle of the internal os is damaged, there may be problems during pregnancy. The internal os stops the baby, which after all

71

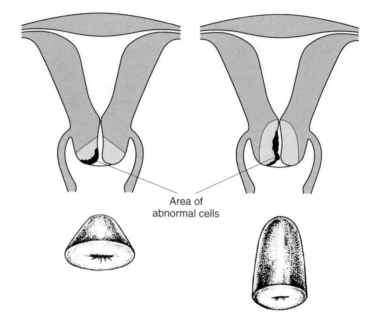

Figure 5.6 'Short' and 'long' cone biopsies.

becomes heavier and heavier, from 'falling out' of the womb before a woman is ready to go into labour. If the muscle becomes weak, the weight of the baby may become too much for it and a miscarriage occurs. Most miscarriages occur early in pregnancy, but if weak muscle is the cause, the miscarriage will usually occur after the third month. In order to stop this happening, a stitch, which resembles a purse-string, can be inserted into the cervix during early pregnancy. This type of stitch is called a Shirodkar suture, after the doctor who first used it. It is removed when the woman reaches the 38th week of pregnancy and she then goes into labour normally. Incidentally, although problems can occur during pregnancy, having a cone biopsy is unlikely to cause any problems with fertility, i.e. with your ability to actually become pregnant.

Nowadays surgical cone biopsies are smaller than they were in the past, because the area of abnormality can be mapped out more accurately using the colposcope. Because of this, the complications described are less likely to occur.

Cone biopsies performed using the laser or loop diathermy

Both the laser and loop diathermy are now used to perform cone biopsies, and these have advantages over the surgical procedure. When a laser beam is made very narrow, the energy is so concentrated that the beam becomes equivalent to a knife: instead of just evaporating cells away, it will cut through tissue. Laser cone biopsies are more accurate and therefore remove less tissue than surgical cone biopsies. Because the laser beam is such a sharp, clean 'knife' and its heat helps blood vessels seal up quickly, there is less bleeding and less scarring than with surgical cone biopsies. As a result, they are much less likely to result in any of the problems described above.

The loop diathermy can be used for cone biopsies very simply by choosing a larger size wire loop. Otherwise the procedure is much the same as for an ordinary treatment. Indeed, with the advent of loop diathermy, the whole distinction between ordinary treatment and cone biopsy has become slightly blurred; for example, if a woman has severe dyskaryosis on her smear, but nothing can be seen on colposcopy, nowadays it is possible to perform an ordinary loop treatment before resorting to a larger cone biopsy. If the specimen is found to have completely removed the abnormality, nothing further needs to be done. Like laser cones, the loop causes very little scarring and less tissue is removed than with surgical cone biopsies, so there are fewer long-term complications.

Both laser and loop diathermy cone biopsies can be performed under a local anaesthetic in the outpatient clinic, which is another advantage over the surgical procedure. However, the feasibility will depend on how large the cone biopsy needs to be, how easy it is to see your cervix and how nervous you are. They do take longer than ordinary treatments, so some women prefer a general anaesthetic. However, both types are less likely to cause problems with bleeding, so many women can go home the same day. Of course, all the advice given earlier about your activities after treatment applies with even greater force under these circumstances.

What happens after a cone biopsy?

The piece of your cervix is sent to a laboratory, where it is examined in detail. Your doctor will want to know not just what degree of abnormality was present, but also whether it has been completely removed, i.e. whether the edges of the piece were clear of abnormal cells. The results usually take about 2 weeks; some doctors ask you to come back to discuss them, or you may be notified by letter.

If there was no suggestion of early cancer, and the abnormality was completely removed, you will be seen usually 4–9 months after the treatment, for a colposcopy and smear. Then, if everything is fine, you may be asked simply to have yearly smears, or the doctor may want to see you for colposcopy once more, in 6–12 months, just to be on the safe side.

If the abnormality was not completely removed by the cone biopsy, you may be followed up more frequently in the colposcopy clinic, in case another treatment becomes necessary. Often, the remaining abnormal cells go away without further treatment, so it is worth watching and waiting for a while.

Another important part of the laboratory examination of the cone biopsy is to check whether it shows any signs of early cancer. Cancerous cells want to spread, so they push through the basement membrane, which normally keeps the outer layers of cells separated from the deeper tissues. The basement membrane has already been mentioned in Chapter 1 and I will go into greater detail about the spread of early cancer in Chapter 6. If there has only been a very slight spread, the cancer is described as microinvasive; if it has been completely removed by the cone biopsy, no further treatment is likely to be needed, though obviously you will be monitored carefully. However, if there has been more extensive spread, further treatment will be required. All this is dealt with more fully in Chapter 6.

Why do some women have a hysterectomy when they only have abnormal cells, not cancer?

Hysterectomy, or removal of the womb (uterus) is sometimes advised when there is another reason for doing it anyway. For example, if you also have very heavy periods, or fibroids (swellings of the muscle in the womb) and you have completed your family, a hysterectomy would solve all the problems at once. Indeed, it would be pretty pointless to have treatment to your cervix, only to have the whole womb removed a few months later. However, a hysterectomy is a big operation, requiring a stay in hospital for a week, several weeks off work and it is often 2 months before you feel fully recovered. You should therefore have thought the decision through very carefully and discussed it thoroughly with your gynaecologist before going ahead.

If a woman has cervical cancer, her hysterectomy is likely to be performed in a different way from the 'normal' type. This is discussed in Chapter 6.

6 CERVICAL CANCER AND ITS TREATMENT

So far in this book I have dealt with conditions (i.e. abnormal cells) that, although they may have the potential to become cancer in the future, are in themselves quite harmless. This chapter looks briefly at 'real' cervical cancer and how it is diagnosed and treated. In practice, a diagnosis of cervical cancer is rare in this country: at present around 3000 women each year develop it. This compares with between 200 000 and 300 000 women who have some kind of abnormality on their smear.

One of the difficulties in discussing cervical cancer is that every woman with cancer will have a different disease pattern, different circumstances and different individual considerations. Thus, the best person to ask for information and advice is your own gynaecologist, who knows the details of your case. Other people (even other doctors), friends and books can never give you specific advice and may actually be misleading.

Thus, this chapter is simply intended as a guide, to help you understand the basics. Then hopefully, you will be better equipped to ask questions and make sense of the often quite complicated answers.

How will I know if I have cervical cancer?

I always thought you'd only need to go for a smear if there was something wrong. So when I started to get bleeding, often after we'd made love, I went to my doctor. He started to do the smear, but then said he'd send me straight to the hospital.

I just went along for my 5-yearly smear. I'd never had any problems before. I guessed something was wrong because the doctor rang me to come and discuss my result.

Unfortunately, you normally don't notice anything wrong until you already have cancer. This is why regular smears are important, even though everything feels fine.

There are a few signs to look out for, but all of these are more commonly due to something other than cancer. Unusual bleeding can be a warning sign, perhaps between periods, after sex, or suddenly for no reason after periods have completely stopped at the menopause (change of life). However, bleeding after sex is very often simply due to an ectopy (see Chapter 3), which is a harmless condition. Bleeding between periods can occur in women who use an intrauterine device (IUD) for contraception. Some women get a little spotting mid-cycle when they ovulate.

Women taking the combined oral contraceptive pill can have what is known as 'breakthrough bleeding', meaning bleeding on days when they are still taking pills. This can be caused by forgetting pills, taking interacting medication such as antibiotics, or having a stomach upset. If persistent, a change of brand should help. In any case of unusual bleeding, the doctor may first want to examine you and check whether you are up to date with your smears,

Vaginal discharge may be a warning sign of cancer, but, of course, by far the most common reason is an infection. An ectopy can also sometimes cause discharge (see Chapter 3).

In the majority of cases of early cancer, women have not noticed anything unusual. The only way to prevent it happening to you is by regular screening.

Squamous cell cancer and adenocarcinoma

There are two types of cervical cancer. By far the most common, accounting for around 90% of cases, is squamous cell cancer. This arises from the flat squamous cells, usually in the area of the transformation zone (see Chapter 1). When people talk about cervical cancer, this is the type they usually mean.

Adenocarcinoma ('carcinoma' is just another word for 'cancer') arises from the endocervical, columnar cells. It is rare; only around 10% of cancers are of this type (and cervical cancer of any kind is not common in this country). It is much harder to detect by screening, as the cells are more difficult to pick up (they are more likely to be hidden inside the cervical canal) and also to recognise under the microscope. Indeed, screening is really designed to pick up the squamous cell abnormalities rather than these much, much rarer columnar cell ones. We still do not know a great deal about adenocarcinoma, either its causes or its management. It may be on the increase, as the number of cases seems to be rising, but that may be partly due to the fact that doctors are becoming better at recognising it. It is still a grey area and in this book I shall only discuss squamous cell cancer in more detail, though the treatment for both types is similar.

How far has the cancer progressed?

Cervical cancer is described in terms of stages, or degrees of severity. These stages are useful for a couple of reasons. First, it means that different treatments can be compared fairly, since the chances of success are likely to be greater the earlier a cancer is found. Second, it means that a woman can be given a reasonable idea of what her chances are, based on experience of other women who have had cancer of similar severity.

I am not going to go into great depth about the staging, since it is quite complicated and involves a detailed knowledge of anatomy. There are four stages, with each stage being further subdivided into two others, called a and b. The idea is to describe how far the cancer cells have spread. In a Stage 1 cancer, only the womb itself is involved. A Stage 2 cancer has spread just outside the womb, for example to involve part of the vagina. In Stage 3, the cancer is still contained within the pelvis, but only just. Stage 4 means the cancer cells have spread outside the pelvis, to the bladder, the bowel, or to more distant organs like the lungs and the liver.

How do cancer cells spread?

In very early cancer, the cells simply increase in number and push away or squash the normal cells. This is called microinvasion (see below). At this point it is still possible to remove the cancer cells by doing a cone biopsy (see Chapter 5), leaving the rest of the cervix and womb intact.

If the cancer cells are not stopped, they will carry on increasing in number and will eventually push their way into the lymph channels. Lymph is a liquid which carries immune cells ('white cells') around the body. These immune cells are a little like policemen on the beat; there are always some around in the lymph channels, but if they sense 'intruders', such as bacteria, viruses or cancer cells, huge numbers will be alerted and rush to the scene.

Unfortunately, these lymph channels can also be used by cancer cells in order to spread around the body. Lymph channels often run alongside blood vessels and constitute a large network, rather like streets in a city. Every now and again there are places where large numbers of immune cells congregate, called lymph nodes. You can think of these as 'police stations', containing large numbers of 'policemen', or immune cells. Cancer cells tend to get trapped inside lymph nodes, just as a criminal would find it hard to escape from a police station. However, they put up a fight, and so lymph nodes containing trapped cancer cells may be swollen and sometimes tender. You can now see why doctors often examine the lymph node areas: although you cannot see cancer cells moving, you can get an idea of whether they have spread by seeing if the lymph nodes have increased in size.

(Incidentally, this swelling and tenderness of the lymph nodes can occur in any condition where the immune cells are fighting an intruder: infections are a much more common cause than cancer. So please do not panic if you unexpectedly find a slightly enlarged lymph node!)

By using lymph channels as if they were roads, cervical cancer cells can gradually spread further and further away from their original site. Eventually they can reach organs as far away as the lungs. Obviously, the further they spread, the more difficult it is to get rid of them. Equally, if they have managed to get so far, they must have defeated the body's immune 'fighting policemen', again reducing the chances of success.

For this reason, if there is any chance that the cancer has spread, tests need to be carried out to check where they might have reached. There is no point just taking out the womb if the lungs are already involved. Not all cancers behave in the same way: some appear to be more aggressive and spread faster than others.

Microinvasion

As its name suggests, microinvasion is the very earliest stage of cancer, often referred to as 1a in the medical staging system.

If you recall the discussion of CIN change in Chapter 2, the important point about CIN is that it does not go through the basement membrane. It is wholly contained on the outside surface of the cervical 'skin'. When invasion starts to occur, the abnormal cells break through the basement

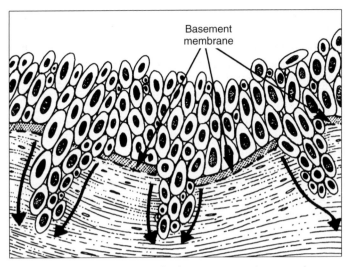

Figure 6.1   Abnormal cells crossing the basement membrane to the connective tissue.

membrane. In microinvasion, the cells can be seen to have only just broken through, and should not have managed to get far enough to reach the lymphatic channels. This is where problems start to occur, because it is difficult to be sure what depth of microinvasion is still 'safe'. If it is 'safe', then the cone biopsy – which is always done if there is a suspicion of microinvasion (see Chapter 5) – will be enough to cure the condition. Otherwise, a hysterectomy will be necessary. This is why the cone biopsy is looked at so carefully under the microscope: the distance the cells have travelled on the 'wrong' side of the basement membrane has to be measured to an accuracy of less than a millimetre.

John and I had only been married 3 months when the smear result came back, just showing abnormal cells. It was only when I went to the hospital that the consultant said I might have early cancer. It was such a shock. He said first of all I should have a cone-shaped piece removed and they would see if that was enough. So I had that done a week later. Actually, it wasn't as bad as I'd thought, it was all over in a few minutes. Waiting for the result was the worst part. It took a week but it felt like years. John went with me to the hospital. The doctor said they probably had removed all the cancer cells, but he couldn't be absolutely sure. He asked if we wanted children. John and I hadn't thought of starting a family quite yet, we had thought we'd wait a couple of years. But we did want children eventually. He said we should talk about it, because it might be better to have a child sooner and then perhaps have the hysterectomy for my protection. He said we shouldn't decide there and then, he'd see us again in a week.

We sat and talked all evening. At first John was so worried about me that he said I should just have the operation and we could always adopt a baby. But I thought it would never be the same as having one of our own. If we tried for a baby straight away, just one, and then I had the hysterectomy afterwards, at least we'd have a child, even if we did adopt a second one. And, in the end, that's what we did. I've been lucky: now I've got Amy and it seems I have been cured. I still go for regular check-ups, but I feel healthy. I think it's going to be OK.

Sometimes, even with all the careful measuring and checking of the tissue, it is still not possible to be absolutely sure that the lymph channels are clear. This is one of the times when a woman's individual circumstances and wishes would influence what was done. If she has completed her family and perhaps has other gynaecological problems, she could opt for what would be the safest course, which would be to have a hysterectomy (removal of the uterus, or womb). However, she may have no children and still wish to have a family. In this case, obviously, it would be very upsetting to have a hysterectomy. She may decide just to have the cone biopsy and be carefully monitored in the colposcopy clinic. This involves a slight risk, but one she may be prepared to take in order to be able to have children.

There is now another option, known as trachelectomy, for women who would in the past have been advised to have a hysterectomy, but are very keen to preserve their fertility. This essentially involves removing virtually the whole of the cervix, but leaves the rest of the womb, thus allowing pregnancy. A stitch is put in around the upper opening of the cervix to hold it closed; this is a permanent stitch, so any baby would have to be delivered by Caesarean section. The operation has been available in some specialist centres for 5–10 years and seems to give a good chance of successful pregnancy. However, there is a significant risk of miscarriage or premature birth because the cervix may not be able to support the weight of the growing pregnancy. Because the procedure has only been carried out in the last 5–10 years, there is relatively little information regarding its success in the treatment of cancer; at present, it appears that 95% of (carefully chosen) women are disease-free 5 years after the operation. As I said at the beginning of this chapter, in such circumstances, you need to discuss things carefully with your gynaecologist.

Invasive cancer

An obviously invasive cancer is more likely to cause symptoms such as bleeding and discharge. In this case, the cone biopsy will reveal that the cancer has spread through to the lymph channels, and therefore potentially to other areas of the body. For this reason, before any treatment is contemplated, tests need to be done to check the organs which might be involved.

The bladder, kidneys and rectum are close to the womb and are therefore obvious places to start. Often, the first thing the gynaecologist will want to do is a full internal examination under general anaesthetic. You may ask: why isn't the one he did while I was awake enough? The reason is that under anaesthetic your muscles are fully relaxed, which makes it easier to perform the examination and gives more information. In addition, the bladder can then be checked directly by passing a flexible tube with a light source into it. This is called a cystoscopy and allows the doctor to actually see inside the bladder and check it for cancer. The same type of thing can be done for the rectum (back passage): not only can an ordinary examination be performed, but again, a special tube can be inserted to allow the doctor to see what is going on higher up.

The kidneys are checked by doing a special type of X-ray called an intravenous pyelogram (IVP) or urogram (IVU). For this, you have a dye injected into a vein in your arm. The dye travels through the bloodstream to the kidneys and can then be photographed while it is passing through the kidneys and bladder. Doctors know what the pictures should look like if there is no abnormality, so they can tell if there is something unusual there.

A chest X-ray is usually done to check there is no cancer in the lungs – and also, it is useful if an operation is being considered. You will have several blood tests, for example to make sure you are not anaemic.

Another test which is sometimes performed is a lymphangiogram. This shows up the lymph nodes and helps predict which ones may have been invaded by the cancer. For this, a special dye is injected into your feet: don't be worried when you and your urine turn green, it does wear off!

There are a number of other special scans and tests (for example magnetic resonance imaging or MRI and computerised tomography or CT scans) that can be done. Whether you have them will depend on whether your gynaecologist feels they are necessary, and, of course, some may simply not be available at your hospital.

When you have had these tests, your gynaecologist will be in a position to discuss the treatment options with you. Once again, what is done will obviously partly depend on what he or she feels is the best form of treatment, but also on your own individual circumstances and wishes. There are two main types of treatment for cervical cancer, which are surgery and radiotherapy. A combination of the two may also be used. In general, doctors try and use surgery for younger women if possible, since this usually allows the ovaries to continue functioning and has fewer long-term complications. Radiotherapy is nowadays also often combined with chemotherapy, as this seems to improve the success of the treatment.

Surgical treatment

This involves a special type of hysterectomy, called a Wertheim's hysterectomy. It is a bigger operation than a normal hysterectomy because the lymph nodes in the pelvic area are also removed. This is done for two reasons. First, removing the lymph nodes will hopefully catch cancer cells 'in transit' and stop them travelling onward. Second, the lymph nodes are looked at in detail under a microscope and, by knowing where they came from, it is possible to tell how far the cancer has spread. This means the doctor can tell with more accuracy how successful the operation is likely to be.

Although the operation is a large one, the ovaries are left behind unless the woman has already gone through the menopause (change of life) anyway. This is good for younger women, since it means they will still have functioning ovaries. However, there is a chance that the ovaries will gradually stop working anyway because their blood supply may have been slightly damaged during the operation. It is important to have blood tests to check the hormone levels occasionally, and especially if you notice hot flushes. If there are signs that the ovaries are running down, hormone replacement therapy can be given.

A Wertheim's hysterectomy is a long operation, often taking several hours. This is partly because of the time required to remove the lymph nodes, but also because it is all too easy to damage the bladder and other nearby organs if great care is not taken.

When you wake up, you will discover that you have a urinary catheter. This is a tube going into your bladder and attached to a bag, to keep your bladder empty. This is necessary because the bladder takes some time to start working properly again after the operation. You will stay in hospital for about 2 weeks after the operation, but most women find that it takes a couple of months before they feel completely back to normal.

By the time you leave hospital, the microscopic examination of the womb and the lymph nodes will have been done, so the doctor will be able to let you know those results and discuss what to do next, if anything. Often just having an operation is enough, but if many lymph nodes are found to contain cancer cells, a course of radiotherapy may be advised as well.

You will be followed up regularly every 3 months or so for the first couple of years and then gradually less frequently until you are seen just once a year. You may be asked not to have sex for the first couple of months after the operation, to allow the area to heal.

Surgery is only possible while the cancer is still fairly early and therefore localised. As I mentioned earlier, it is preferable in young women because the ovaries are preserved and there are fewer long-term complications. However, if the cancer has spread beyond the pelvic area, thus being too advanced for surgery, or if surgical treatment is not successful in removing all of the cancer, radiotherapy may be better. This may also be the case in older women or those who for various reasons are not suitable for surgical treatment.

Radiotherapy

There are two types of radiotherapy that can be used, internal and external. The cervix is relatively unusual, in that it is accessible enough for internal radiotherapy.

Internal radiotherapy involves the insertion of radioactive rods inside the uterus and vagina. The advantage of this is that the cervix and uterus (womb) receive quite a high dose of radiation, but the bladder, bowel and rectum receive much less, because they are further away. This minimises the side effects of the treatment, described below.

Internal radiotherapy is a lonely procedure because you emit radiation while you are having it, so you have to be kept in a room on your own for a couple of days. However, you do not usually need more than three treatments, several days, or even a week apart. The treatment itself does not hurt; most women complain more of boredom and being stiff from lying still.

Internal radiotherapy can be used on its own if the cancer is still fairly early, but the more advanced types require external treatment, to cover a larger area.

External radiotherapy involves short treatments spread over 3–6 weeks. It is rather like lying on a sunbed and you can talk to the staff, who will be behind a protective screen. You usually have to come for the treatment several days each week, which is one of its most tiresome aspects. You have to keep travelling to and fro, all for a treatment which lasts a few minutes at a time. Since nausea and diarrhoea are common side effects, this travelling is not the trivial thing you would first suppose.

Internal and external radiotherapy are usually used in combination. External radiotherapy may also be used in combination with surgery, either to shrink the tumour before the operation, or afterwards, to clear any remaining cancer away.

During either type of radiotherapy, the main problem is that, despite shielding, organs that are not the focus of the treatment get irradiated anyway. In particular, this affects the bladder and the bowel. Diarrhoea and nausea are common, but can be made more bearable by using medication. Symptoms that resemble cystitis may occur, but these usually get better.

The vagina and ovaries are also affected. The ovaries will stop working, so you are likely to be given hormone replacement therapy afterwards. The vagina shrinks and becomes less elastic, partly as a direct effect of the radiation, but also because of the loss of the oestrogen hormone from the ovaries. Following radiotherapy, it is important to try and have sex quite soon, or the shrinkage can become permanent. This is another reason why radiotherapy is generally avoided in young women.

Chemotherapy together with radiotherapy

As its name suggests, chemotherapy involves treatment using chemicals, given either by mouth or by injection. They are also called 'cytotoxics' ('cyto' means 'cell') because they kill cells. Unfortunately, they tend to lack discrimination and kill normal as well as abnormal cells, so they often have unpleasant side effects. These can include nausea, vomiting and hair loss. In the last few years, research has shown that a combination of radiotherapy and chemotherapy seems to give better results than just radiotherapy alone. It may be that the chemotherapy makes cancer cells more sensitive to the effects of the radiotherapy.

How successful are the treatments?

Specific predictions can only be made by the gynaecologist who is actually dealing with the case. Do not be afraid to ask. In general terms, if the cancer is caught early enough, before the lymph nodes are involved, there is a good chance of cure, around 80–90%. However, if the lymph nodes are already involved and therefore the cancer has managed to spread to other parts of the body, the chance of success is only 50%; this means that half the women who present with later stage cancers die within 5 years. And remember that many of those women will not have noticed anything wrong until it was too late. Once again, let me remind you of the importance of regular screening.

7   WHY ME? THE POSSIBLE CAUSES OF CIN AND CERVICAL CANCER

It has been known for over a century that cervical cancer is closely associated with sexual activity. However, as we shall see, there must be other factors involved.

In 1842, an Italian doctor called Rigoni-Stern noticed that nuns very rarely developed cancer of the cervix. When he looked into this more deeply, he found that not all nuns seemed to be 'immune' – women who had been married before entering the order appeared to be at roughly the same risk as the general population. He concluded that virginity must be the protective factor.

Sexual behaviour

Rigoni-Stern's work was largely ignored for over a hundred years, until a Canadian doctor repeated the study, looking at nuns in Quebec. This opened the floodgates of research into this area in the 1950s. Suddenly everyone was interested in cervical cancer. Within a few years it had been established that the disease was particularly common in prostitutes and that a very important risk factor was the age at which a woman first had sex. Indeed, it has been found that women who start having sex below the age of 17 years have more than twice the risk of those who start after the age of 20. Also, the more partners a woman had, the greater her risk: women with four partners had twice the risk of those who only had one.

Soon it was found that young age at first pregnancy placed a woman at risk, while women with few or no pregnancies seemed less at risk than those who had many pregnancies. Divorced, widowed or separated women were at risk. It was even discovered that women who attended church regularly were less likely to develop the disease than their non-attending counterparts.

Scientists started to look at the differences in incidence in various countries, and found them to be quite striking. Colombia had an incidence nearly 100 times greater than that of Israel; the USA and Europe were somewhere in-between. Then they looked at different ethnic groups. It was interesting that Jewish women tended to have the same incidence regardless of which country they lived in. The scientists then compared Jewish women, white Americans and non-white Americans who all lived in the same place, New York. Non-white American women had the highest incidence, Jewish women the lowest and white Americans were in-between.

Next, it was noticed that there was a difference between the social classes, and also within each social class. At that time (and often to this day), social class grading was usually done according to the occupation of the husband. It was found that there was a much higher incidence of cervical cancer in the lower social classes. However, regardless of social class, there was a higher incidence among women married to men whose jobs involved travel and long periods away from home, for example sailors, long-distance lorry drivers, soldiers and so on. Table 7.1 shows you how the risks varied according to the husband's occupation.

So the doctors and scientists looked at all these pieces of information and tried to find something that would link them together. The conclusion seemed inescapable: it must relate to the woman's sexual behaviour. What do prostitutes, widows, divorced women, women who marry very young or start having sex very young, have in common? They are likely to have more than one sexual partner in their lifetime. So started the 'cervical cancer is a disease of promiscuity' story. Nuns have no sexual partners, Jewish and very religious women of any denomination tend to have only one partner – it all seemed to fit.

Then a few little contradictions started to creep in. How come cervical cancer was very common in upper social class women in Colombia, who were usually faithful to their husbands? And who was more likely to have large numbers of sexual partners, the sailor or his wife? In the late 1960s the attention therefore turned to men.

An important study looked at men whose first wives had died of cervical cancer. It was found that their subsequent wives were nearly three times as likely to develop the disease. The sexual behaviour of men in Colombia was then studied, and it was found that the well-to-do Colombian man was accustomed to visiting prostitutes on a regular basis, while his wife remained faithful. A further study looked specifically at

Table 7.1 Risk of cervical cancer by social class and husband's occupation in married women (England and Wales 1959–63)

Social class	Occupation of husband	Woman's risk of cervical cancer*
I	All occupations	34
	Clergymen	12
	Scientists	17
	Civil engineers	60
II	All occupations	64
	Teachers	30
	Senior government officials	40
	Publicans and innkeepers	120
	Lodging house and hotel keepers	150
III	All occupations	100
	Clerks of work	40
	Clerks	64
	Crane and hoist operators	159
	Drivers of road goods vehicles	168
IV	All occupations	116
	Shopkeepers and assistants	71
	Gardeners and groundsmen	98
	Fishermen	257
	Boatmen	263

*Higher number equals higher risk.

men, to see how the numbers of partners influenced their wives' risk of cervical cancer (the wives in the study all said they had had only one partner, their husband). If the man had had more than 15 partners, his wife's risk of developing cervical cancer was nearly eight times greater than if he had only had one partner. All these studies led to the concept of the 'high-risk male', which is discussed in greater detail in the next chapter.

So it was not just the sexual behaviour of women that was important – the behaviour of men had to be taken into account as well. On the basis of the new findings, three models of behaviour were drawn up to try to explain the differences in incidence between different countries, ethnic groups and religious denominations (see Figure 7.1).

In a type A society both the woman and the man have only one sexual partner, i.e. each other. This is the type of behaviour found amongst religious Jews and certain other religious denominations. The incidence of cervical cancer is very low.

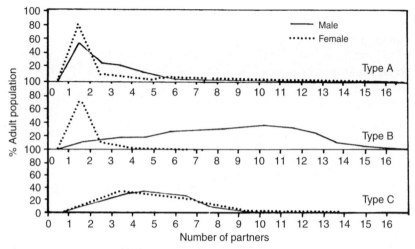

Figure 7.1 Patterns of behaviour in three types of society.

In a type B society, the woman has only one partner, but the man has many. This was the case in Colombia and also in Victorian England. The incidence of cervical cancer is very high.

In a type C society both the man and the woman have more than one partner, but neither has a large number of partners. This is the general pattern of behaviour in Europe and the USA today. The incidence of cervical cancer is above that of type A, but well below that of type B societies.

Other suspected factors

Having established that cervical cancer was in some way related to sex, the next obvious question was: 'What is it that passes between a man and a woman to cause the disease?' And it did not take long for people to start looking at sperm. It has been shown that sperm can become attached to the very cells on the cervix that can eventually become abnormal. Certain types of protein, which are part of the sperm head, may be able to interfere in some way with the functions of the cell. In addition, sperm may be able to reduce the immune (defensive) response of the cervical cells. The exact mechanisms for these effects are unknown, and they are certainly weak; however, it is possible that they 'help' some other agent to cause abnormalities in the cells. This is known as being a 'cofactor', and we will come across this concept again later. One study has also shown that the human papillomavirus (which is discussed in Chapter 8) can be passed on through semen.

The next suggestion was that it might be something to do with personal hygiene. This was based mainly on the fact that there was a low incidence amongst Jewish women, whose partners are circumcised. Perhaps smegma, the substance that collects under the foreskin, had something to do with it? The idea of personal hygiene seemed to tie in well with the social class variation. A man coming home after a long day's work at the coal face might well be more 'dirty' than an office clerk. Unfortunately for this theory, the facts just did not add up. For example, there is a tribe in Malaysia that still lives in a very primitive fashion. The men are uncircumcised, the girls marry at about the age of 14 and they have never heard of the idea of hygiene. In addition the women start having children immediately after their marriage and tend to have a large number (they haven't heard of contraception either). Despite all this, their incidence of cervical cancer is very low. Of more significance is the fact that they do not have premarital sex, and remain faithful to each other after marriage. And, of course, this is also the more likely explanation for the low incidence of cervical cancer amongst Jews. In this context, it is interesting to note that more recent work suggests that the incidence of cervical cancer in non-orthodox Jewish women is rising: Jewish men are still usually circumcised, whether orthodox or not, but presumably the main difference lies in a less strict code of sexual behaviour.

Smoking

In recent years, smoking has become a focus of attention. An association between smoking and cervical cancer was noticed as long ago as 1977, but at first it was dismissed as being improbable – after all, how does the smoke get all the way down to the cervix? And maybe it was just that women who smoked were also more likely to have sex young and have more partners. However, even when those factors were taken into account, smokers still appeared to be at greater risk than non-smokers. The exact degree of the increase in risk varies from study to study, but the risk of actual cancer appears to be increased by about a factor of two, and that of CIN 3 (the third stage of abnormal cells) by up to 12 times.

Then, in the 1980s, several studies showed that components of cigarette smoke, including nicotine and cotinine, were actually found in high concentrations in cervical mucus. The amounts were even higher than in the blood of the same women, so it looked as though, for some reason, these potentially cancer-producing substances were congregating around the cervix. Thus, suddenly, there was an obvious way in which smoking could be contributing to the risk of cervical cancer.

There is another way in which smoke-related poisons might be involved, by reducing the immune defence mechanisms of the cervical cells. Studies have shown that the number of special immune cells in the cervix, called Langerhans cells (after a doctor called Paul Langerhans) is reduced in women who have CIN. There are several other types of immune cell that can be similarly affected. It has also been shown that these immune cells are reduced in number in women who smoke. Thus, the same thing happens in both cases. If there are fewer immune cells, the cervical cells are less able to defend themselves against attackers. Thus, smoking may help some other, probably sexually transmitted agent, to cause cervical cancer. Once again, it may be acting as a cofactor.

A study has shown that women with early cervical abnormalities can help themselves get better by stopping smoking. This is quite exciting, because it suggests that even if you have a mildly abnormal smear, there is still the opportunity to get rid of the abnormal cells by giving up smoking, rather than having treatment. There is, however, no evidence that giving up will make more severely abnormal cells get better; by then they have probably gone beyond the point of no return.

Diet

In the last 10 years there has been some suggestion that a diet deficient in certain vitamins may increase the risk of cervical cancer. However, the picture is still rather unclear, with studies giving conflicting results, both as to whether vitamins are involved at all and also as to which vitamins may be important. The ones that may be of interest are vitamin C, vitamin E and beta-carotene, which is part of vitamin A. These vitamins have something in common: they all 'mop up' free radicals, which are nasty substances, thought to be involved in a number of cancers. Thus, the idea that they may be useful is plausible. However, it is possible that only a severe deficiency is important; the studies suggesting a link have tended to be from the developing world, in areas where diet is very poor.

So far, there is no evidence that taking extra vitamin supplements is of any use, either in prevention or cure, but since no-one has any idea of the possible doses needed, studies have not been very satisfactory. It is in any case a minefield in which to try and do research. Measuring people's intake of vitamins is fraught with problems: questionnaires may not be representative of a person's diet, may not be filled in properly, or may be misunderstood. Blood tests are quite expensive, difficult to do and in any case not popular. There are so many other things that could affect blood levels: for example, it is known that smokers who eat the same amount of vitamins as non-smokers have lower blood levels. Presumably, smokers do not absorb their vitamins as well. And we have seen that smoking may in any case increase the risk of cancer.

At present it is impossible to be sure what effect, if any, vitamins may have. Research is continuing, but I doubt whether there will be definite answers for some time.

Contraception

Studies looking at contraceptive use and cervical cancer are rather obviously hampered by the fact that the majority of people use contraception when they are having sex. And since sex itself seems to be the most important risk factor, it is difficult to separate the effects of one from the other. In addition, it is possible that people choosing different methods of contraception also behave differently – they may have different numbers of partners, different smoking habits and so on.

However, if the main cause of cervical cancer is a sexually transmitted agent, then one would expect barrier methods of contraception to be protective and, indeed, this does appear to be the case. Use of both diaphragms and condoms is associated with a reduced risk of cervical cancer. Interestingly, the use of spermicides alone (for example foams) also appears to reduce the risk. Spermicides are designed to kill or immobilise sperm, but can also have some effect on bacteria, possibly even on viruses.

Intrauterine contraceptive devices (IUDs) and progestogen-only methods of contraception (pills, injections, implants) do not appear to have any effect on cervical cancer risk.

The relationship between use of the combined oral contraceptive pill and the risk of cervical cancer remains controversial. Here we come across two pitfalls: first, the usual one of other known risk factors confusing the issue, but second, the fact the formulation of the pill has been changing during the last 30 years. Until the mid-1980s studies looking at pill use and the risk of cervical cancer did not take smoking history into account. Nowadays, women taking the pill are advised not to smoke, mainly because of the risk of heart disease. However, when the pill was first introduced, the risks of smoking in relation to pill use and heart disease were not appreciated. Indeed, these high-dose pills were being handed out even to women smokers who were over 35 years old, right up to the early 1980s. It was only then that the risks of heart disease became apparent, and it was also around then that the link between smoking and cervical cancer became established.

In the 1960s and 1970s, for a woman to be on the pill was daring and liberated; so was smoking. It is therefore not too surprising that pill users were actually more likely to smoke than were users of other contraceptive methods. Since smokers have been shown to have more sexual partners than non-smokers, there would be a relatively higher proportion of pill users also in this category. We have already seen that the number of sexual partners is an important risk factor in its own right. I am sure you can already see that all this makes trying to look at pill use on its own very difficult.

The dose of hormones in the pill has been coming down progressively during the last 30 years. Not only that, but the hormones themselves have been modified. Low-dose pills have been around since the early 1980s, but the newest pills only since the mid- to late 1980s. Research studies take many years to conduct and to analyse; how do we know whether the results of studies looking at women using older, high-dose pills are relevant to women today?

A recent study from developing countries managed to get around some (but not all) of the problems associated with differing sexual behaviour patterns. They found no increase in the risk of cervical cancer for use of the pill of less than 5 years. For use of between 5 and 9 years, there did seem to be an increase in risk, but it disappeared within 6 years of stopping the pill. However, again, although the study did suggest that long-term users of the pill may be at greater risk of cervical cancer, it does not prove that the pill actually causes cervical cancer.

It is possible that the pill may act as a 'helper' to some other, sexually transmitted agent. Even then, its effect would be weaker than that of smoking. It is also important to remember that the pill is an extremely effective contraceptive, giving 99% protection against pregnancy. Pregnancy can be a cause of a number of health problems, not only as a possible risk factor for cervical cancer.

What, then, should be the advice for a pill user today? Well, the most obvious thing is to have regular smears; this is the single most important action you can take, regardless of your method of contraception. If you are very worried about cervical cancer, a 'belt and braces' approach would be to use a barrier method in addition to the pill. Although barriers may protect your cervix, remember they are not as effective as the pill in terms of contraception.

Even if you have an abnormal smear, even if you have to have treatment, you can carry on taking the pill. Remember that there is no definite evidence that the pill is implicated in increasing the risk of cervical cancer. It may yet all turn out to have been due to incomplete adjustment for other risk factors. In addition, there is no evidence to suggest that use of the pill makes an abnormal smear get worse, or makes a recurrence more likely.

Deficiencies of the immune system

The immune system is the body's defence mechanism against foreign invaders, whether they are infections or cancers. One would therefore expect that if cervical cancer is primarily due to a sexually transmitted agent, women who for some reason have an impaired immune system would be more likely to develop it.

We have already seen that smoking may reduce the number of immune cells in the cervix and that smokers are at greater risk of developing cervical cancer. Studies have looked at women whose immune systems are depressed for other reasons. For example, women who have kidney transplants have to take strong medication to suppress their immune system, otherwise they will reject their new kidney as a 'foreign invader'. These women have been found to be at increased risk of a number of cancers, including cervical cancer.

Women who are being treated for other cancers using chemotherapy have also been studied. These drugs are potent cell poisons and are known to depress the immune system; once again, such women are at higher risk of developing cervical cancer.

The human immunodeficiency virus (HIV) which causes acquired immune deficiency syndrome (AIDS) is an obvious cause of reduced immunity, and indeed, HIV-positive women have been shown to be more likely to have CIN. However, a problem with looking at HIV-positive women is that they are likely to have other risk factors for cervical cancer. A recent study is interesting, because it compared HIV-negative women attending a department of genito-urinary medicine with HIV-positive women in the same department. Some of the HIV-positive women were perfectly healthy, while others were already beginning to develop AIDS-related illnesses. They found that there was no difference in terms of CIN between the HIV-negative women and the healthy HIV-positive women. However, the HIV-positive women who were showing signs of immune deficiency were more likely to have CIN.

Pregnancy and adolescence

Women who become pregnant young and who have several pregnancies appear to be more at risk of cervical cancer, though partly this effect is due to having had sex under the age of 20. Nevertheless, pregnancy may be a risk factor in its own right.

Pregnancy is another time when the immune system is relatively suppressed. After all, the growing baby is really a 'foreign body' and needs to be protected from destruction by the immune system. It is therefore not altogether surprising that women who have had several pregnancies may be more likely to develop cervical cancer. It used to be thought that CIN also progressed faster during pregnancy, but it may be that the pregnant cervix simply looks worse than it really is.

Pregnancy and adolescence do have something in common. During both, a great deal of activity goes on in the transformation zone. As you will remember from Chapter 2, it is in this area that soft columnar cells change to become tough squamous cells – squamous metaplasia. This is a perfectly normal process, but it is at this time that cells are most vulnerable to any outside influences that might cause them to develop in an abnormal way. During both pregnancy and adolescence, squamous metaplasia goes on at a much faster rate and involves a larger number of cells. This means that there are more cells around that are vulnerable to attack.

Viruses

In the 1960s, scientists everywhere were searching for a sexually transmitted 'agent' that could be the cause of cervical cancer. The idea of viruses being a cause of cancer was one that had long been popular, so it was not surprising that attention soon turned to them. Chapter 8 deals with this, perhaps most significant, part of the story.

8 THE ROLE OF VIRUSES

What is a virus?

Louis Pasteur and his pupil, Emile Roux, were the first scientists to show that something even smaller than bacteria could cause disease in both animals and man. Their work on the rabies virus in the 1880s paved the way for years of intensive research into viruses. The microscopes used at that time were not powerful enough to show up any kind of virus, so these micro-organisms were, in effect, invisible. Scientists could only guess at what they might be like.

There was only one way to study the effects of a virus; a solution made from diseased tissue was passed through a very fine filter, with holes so small that no ordinary cells or bacteria could pass through. This filtered solution was then injected into an animal; the animal still developed the disease, showing that a disease-causing agent had remained in the solution after it was filtered.

This was a big step forward, but they still did not know what it was about the solutions that caused disease. The major breakthrough did not come until 1935, when an American scientist, Wendell Stanley, managed to form crystals from a solution. When he redissolved the crystals in water, they still caused disease. This made it look as though viruses were not alive at all, but just complicated proteins.

The next advance was the discovery that viruses contained either RNA (ribonucleic acid) or DNA (deoxyribonucleic acid). As their names suggest, these substances are found in the nucleus of a cell. They are the building blocks of genes, which can be inherited and code for different types of cells.

A virus uses its own DNA or RNA to take over control of the cell, rather like a terrorist hijacking an aeroplane. It will override the cell's own DNA or RNA and thus use the cell to reproduce itself. However, some viruses may simply enter the cell and lie dormant for long periods of time; this is true of the human papillomavirus (HPV), which I shall be discussing in detail later. Viruses cannot function without a host cell to provide for their needs; in this they are different from bacteria, which are self-sufficient.

The immune response

Viruses are foreign invaders and the body responds by producing an army. White blood cells immediately start manufacturing special proteins that are actually designed specifically to fight a particular virus type. This is rather like having an inbuilt system that can work out what is in a poison and then produce the antidote. These special proteins are called antibodies and travel in the bloodstream to wherever they are needed, rather like an army. This forms the basis of immunity.

Once the body has produced a particular antibody, it retains the 'blueprint' for future reference. Thus, if the same virus tries to invade again, the correct antibody can be produced much more quickly. The body's defence is therefore stronger and the virus has less chance of 'winning'.

Each virus will trigger the manufacture of an antibody type which is very specific to itself. This means the body has to produce a new variety of antibody every time a new type of virus comes along. You will almost

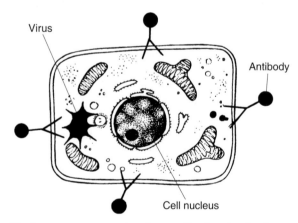

Figure 8.1 The immune response involves antibodies that latch on to a cell after a virus has invaded it.

100

certainly have noticed that having 'flu' once does not seem to protect you from getting it again next year: this is because it is a different kind of 'flu' virus and so there is no 'instant army' waiting to protect you. However, if you have had, say, chicken pox you are very unlikely to get it again because the body will recognise the virus when you come in contact with it once more.

Vaccines are also based on this principle. A vaccine is designed to stimulate the body to produce antibodies against a particular virus or bacterium, so that it will have a ready army when the 'real thing' comes along. The vaccine itself is very similar to the virus, but has been made harmless, like a cobra which has had its fangs removed.

Once a 'blueprint' has been created, small numbers of the specific antibodies circulate in the blood even when there is no infection. This is the way in which your immunity can be checked; for example, a blood test can prove whether you are immune to German measles (rubella), by seeing whether you already have the correct antibodies. This is an important concept, which I shall mention again later.

Viruses and cancer

At first, scientists only looked to see if viruses caused infectious diseases, like bacteria, but in 1911 another French scientist, Rous, demonstrated that a filtered solution could produce cancer in birds. This was the beginning of what proved to be a rapidly expanding area of research. Indeed, people began to think that viruses were the cause of *all* cancers.

Numerous examples of viral cancers started to be found in animals. A virus was found to cause leukaemia in cats, another to cause skin cancer in rabbits, yet another to cause breast cancer in mice. The list is long and continues to grow. Human cancers increasingly became associated with viruses. For example, the virus that causes a type of glandular fever may occasionally also cause cancer of the nasal passages and a type of lymphoma (cancer of the lymph nodes). Another example is provided by one of the viruses that cause hepatitis and which can also cause liver cancer.

It seemed obvious, therefore, to search for a viral cause of cervical cancer. In fact, viruses of several kinds are not too difficult to find in cervical cancer or in CIN (cervical intra-epithelial neoplasia, or abnormal cells, see Chapter 2). The problem is to show that they are not just 'innocent bystanders'. This is an important distinction; by way of analogy, just

101

because someone happens to be found at the scene of a crime does not automatically mean he is guilty of murder.

There have been three main contenders for the role of the 'cervical cancer virus'. These are the human papillomavirus (HPV), herpes simplex virus (HSV) and cytomegalovirus (CMV).

Cytomegalovirus (CMV)

This is a very common virus. It may cause a flu-like illness, or even, occasionally, a type of glandular fever, but most people are quite unaware that they have had the infection. If caught during pregnancy it can be dangerous, because it can affect the baby (rather like German measles).

CMV can also be sexually transmitted and has been found in tissue from the cervix, as well as in semen. This fact led to suspicion that it might be a cause of cervical cancer. Indeed, it was found to be present more often in cervical cancer than in normal tissue. However, it is so common that it is difficult to explain why more women have not developed cancer. It is also quite possible that, once cells have become weakened by the real cancer agent, CMV makes the most of an easy opportunity to invade. It seems unlikely that CMV will prove to be important in the causation of cervical cancer.

Herpes simplex virus (HSV)

This virus has had a troubled career. In the late 1960s, HSV shot to prominence and enjoyed nearly a decade of being 'the' virus. Then, in the 1980s it was denounced as a fraud and sank into obscurity. However, in the last few years it has made a modest comeback, with renewed interest in its possible role.

There are two kinds of herpes virus, HSV 1, which usually causes cold sores, and HSV 2, which usually causes genital herpes (just to complicate matters, they can occasionally swap over). Most interest has centred around HSV 2.

The herpes virus was already known to be capable of causing kidney tumours in frogs. In addition, it is a close relative of the glandular fever virus (the Epstein–Barr virus), which is associated with two types of cancer in humans. Around 1966 it was noticed that women who suffered from genital herpes seemed to have more than their fair share of abnormal smears. Scientists therefore started looking for antibodies to HSV 2 in women with cervical cancer. (Antibodies are explained in detail earlier in this chapter. If a person has antibodies to a virus in their blood, it means that at some point they have been infected with that virus. It is like a fingerprint left behind long after the culprit has gone.) The scientists found that a high proportion of women with cervical cancer had these antibodies, while a group of women who were similar, but did not have cervical cancer, were much less likely to have such antibodies. This looked very promising.

Unfortunately, later studies did not always agree. The proportion of women with cervical cancer who had antibodies to HSV 2 could vary from as high as 90% to as low as 30%. Herpes is a highly infectious disease, and it was quite possible that these figures simply reflected the level of infection in a given area. The studies were, after all, being done during the 'swinging sixties' and early 1970s, when liberated attitudes resulted in an increase in all forms of sexually transmitted disease.

In the 1970s, researchers started to look at the activity of viruses after they had actually got inside the cells. As mentioned earlier, viruses are made up of genetic material, in the form of DNA or RNA; some viruses incorporate their own DNA into that of the cell and in this way the cell's 'instructions' are changed and the virus takes control. However, when scientists looked at cells that had been attacked by the herpes virus, they found that very little, if any, of this incorporation had taken place. The virus seemed to have damaged the cells in various ways, but did not appear to have taken control. It seemed that the herpes virus was behaving in a 'hit and run' fashion. This made it much less likely that the herpes virus could be an important cause of cervical cancer on its own. However, by damaging the cells, it might make them more vulnerable to any further attack, so it might act as a 'primer' for a more important agent.

It is this role that has become of more interest in the last few years. A study has looked at the risk of cervical cancer in women who had HSV 2, human papillomavirus (HPV; see below) or both together. The women who only had HSV 2 showed very little increase in their risk of cervical cancer, while those who only had HPV did have an increased risk. However, there was a quite dramatic effect in the women who had both types of virus: these women were twice as likely to have cervical cancer as those who had the HPV on its own. This suggests that the two viruses interact, with the herpes virus helping the HPV in some way. This is discussed again later.

Having mentioned it, let us now look at HPV. When scientists began to be disillusioned with the herpes theory, they started to notice that the wart, or human papillomavirus (HPV) was often found in cervical cancer tissue. Could this be the virus they had been looking for?

The human papillomavirus (HPV)

It had been known since 1907 that skin warts could be transmitted by a cell-free solution, i.e. by some sort of submicroscopic infective agent. Then, in 1933, it was shown that a wart (correctly called a papilloma virus) caused skin cancer in cotton-tail rabbits. However, an interesting feature which emerged was that the papilloma virus did not always cause cancer; it seemed to need 'help' from some other source. For example, a papilloma virus causes gut cancer in cows, but only if they also eat bracken. Sheep infected with papilloma virus can get skin cancer, but only in parts of the body that are directly exposed to sunlight.

In the late 1970s, workers started to look at cells that had been infected with the papilloma virus and they found that there was not just one papilloma virus, but many different types, which could be identified by the type of DNA they contained. Although they were all related, they seemed to behave quite differently; for example, the type which causes plantar warts (the common verruca) shows little interest in infecting cervical cells. In addition, while some types of papilloma virus could be found in cervical cells, not all of them were actually incorporated into the cells' DNA, so again it appeared that some were just 'innocent bystanders'.

As research technology became more sophisticated, it was possible to work out the exact types of papilloma virus that were present in different places. Currently there are over 100 different types of papilloma virus and the number identified is growing all the time. Type 1 is the verruca virus. The genital warts that you can see on the vulva or the penis are usually caused by HPV types 6 or 11. These are often also found in cervical cells, but they are not incorporated into the cells' DNA. However, when types such as 16, 18, 31, 33 or 45 are found in cervical cells, they *are* usually incorporated into the DNA, and it is these types that are most often found in cervical cancer.

So it looks as though there are low-risk (i.e. unrelated to cancer) viruses (types 6 and 11) and high-risk viruses (15 types including 16, 18, 31, 33, 45). The trouble is that both low-risk and high-risk types can

104

cause cell changes. It is not possible to tell which is which from a cervical smear or even a biopsy, unless special techniques are used to look at the DNA in the cells.

When a cell is invaded by HPV, characteristic changes can be seen under the microscope. These changes are not actually part of the 'abnormal cell' spectrum and the cells that show signs of HPV infection are called koilocytes. You may see this term used on smear reports, though there is now a category in section 23 for 'wart virus' (see Figure 8.2)

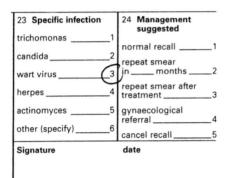

23 Specific infection	24 Management suggested
trichomonas _____1	normal recall _____1
candida _____2	repeat smear
wart virus _____3	in ____ months ____2
herpes _____4	repeat smear after treatment _____3
actinomyces _____5	gynaecological referral _____4
other (specify)_____6	cancel recall _____5
Signature	**date**

Figure 8.2 Section 23 of smear form with 'wart virus' ringed.

A difficulty that often arises is that wart virus (HPV) changes can look similar to abnormal cell changes. In addition, the two can simply occur together. Thus, you are quite likely to see a report of 'borderline dyskaryosis' and 'wart virus change' together (see Figure 8.3).

HPV changes may have a characteristic appearance on colposcopy and may show up in biopsies. The herpes virus can also cause changes in the cells, which may be noted in section 23 of the form.

In addition to changes that can be seen in cells, antibodies are formed to the specific type of papilloma virus or viruses that have caused the infection (see earlier in this chapter) and these antibodies may be detected in blood samples. Studies looking at specific types of HPV have shown that women with cervical cancer are more likely to have antibodies to, for example, HPV type 16, than well women. However, antibody studies are complicated by the large number of HPV types and difficulties with the assays, which are still being refined.

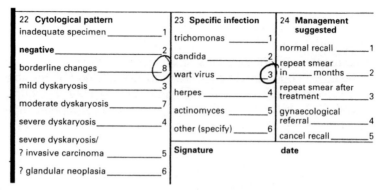

22 Cytological pattern	23 Specific infection	24 Management suggested
inadequate specimen _____1	trichomonas _____1	normal recall _____1
negative_____2	candida _____2	repeat smear
borderline changes_____8	wart virus _____3	in _____ months _____2
mild dyskaryosis _____3	herpes _____4	repeat smear after treatment _____3
moderate dyskaryosis_____7	actinomyces _____5	gynaecological referral _____4
severe dyskaryosis_____4	other (specify) _____6	cancel recall _____5
severe dyskaryosis/ ? invasive carcinoma _____5	Signature	date
? glandular neoplasia_____6		

Figure 8.3 Sections 22 and 23 of smear form showing borderline changes and wart virus.

Evidence for the involvement of the so called 'high-risk' HPV types in CIN and cervical cancer is now overwhelming. HPV has been found in the vast majority (more than 99%) of cervical cancers. What has also become apparent is that although there are 15 HPV types that can potentially cause cervical cancer, some are much more common than others. So types 16 and 18 between them are found in more than 70% of cervical cancers, and are by far the most important (see Figure 8.4).

In recent years it has been shown that the 'high-risk' types of HPV contain special proteins (called E6 and E7), which are able to 'switch on' the transformation process in cells. I have already referred to the fact that the important thing about HPV is its ability to incorporate itself into the cell's DNA and use it for its own purposes. It seems that these E6 and E7 proteins can make a cell 'decide' to grow abnormally. This is rather like a science fiction story in which the enemy alien enters someone's brain and makes that person behave in a way which benefits the alien, perhaps killing comrades, taking over the spaceship and so on.

It also appears that, as in animals, HPV does not cause cancer on its own: it needs help. I have already mentioned that women who are on drugs that suppress their immune response, such as cancer or kidney transplant patients, have been shown to be more likely to develop CIN and cervical cancer (see Chapter 7). The same thing is also true of women who are HIV positive, or have AIDS (also mentioned in the previous chapter). It makes sense that anything that weakens the body's immune system would make it easier for viruses to invade. This also applies to

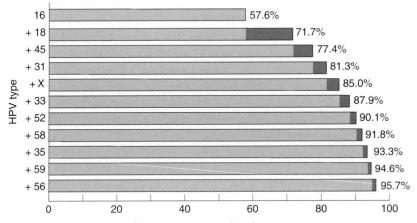

Figure 8.4 Proportion of cancers associated with HPV types.

smoking, which, as we saw in the previous chapter, is now recognised as a risk factor for cervical cancer. Earlier in this chapter, I mentioned a study looking at the interaction between HPV and the herpes virus: it would appear that the herpes virus may be acting as another type of 'helper', or 'cofactor' to allow HPV to invade more easily.

Smoking and herpes are only two possible sources of help for HPV; there may be many others. Sperm proteins, mentioned in Chapter 7, may also act in this way, as may other sexually transmitted infections, such as chlamydia. The necessity for cofactors may well turn out to be the reason why one woman has HPV infection and develops cancer, while another woman can have the same type of HPV but stays well. More research is still needed in this area.

How common is HPV?

HPV is so common that it has been estimated that we have a 75% chance of catching it at some point in our lives. It has been described as 'a natural consequence of having sex'. The important thing is not whether you catch HPV (because you almost certainly will, at some point), but whether your body fights it successfully and you get rid of it. An analogy would be that many people catch colds, but only a small proportion go on to develop a serious chest infection. In most cases, the immune system rallies and eliminates the virus. It is only if this doesn't happen that problems can occur – this is referred to as persistent infection.

As with all infections that are sexually transmitted, HPV is much more common in young people (under 30), in whom it is almost ubiquitous, but almost certainly transient, as mentioned above. If an older woman has HPV, it is more likely that she has had it for longer and has not managed to get rid of it. This is the situation in which HPV can go on to cause cell abnormalities and eventually cancer. I shall come back to this in the context of testing for HPV.

What about men?

So much HPV floating around: but where does it all come from? To answer that question, several studies have been done looking at men. One looked at a group of men whose partners had CIN. Over two-thirds of them were found to have HPV infections of the penis. This fits in well with the concept of the high-risk male, which was first mentioned in Chapter 7. Men may be unaware they have a high-risk HPV infection. The problem, as I mentioned earlier, is that the types that cause visible warts (6 and 11) are not actually the important ones as far as cervical cancer is concerned. It is the invisible ones, for example, HPV types 16, 18, 31, 33 and 45, that are to blame.

Why isn't there an epidemic of penile cancer if so many men are infected? The answer lies in the difference between the cells on the cervix and those on the penis. In Chapter 2, I mentioned that the vulnerable area on the cervix is the transformation zone, where soft columnar cells change into hard, squamous cells. Cells that are in the process of change can be easily attacked by HPV. However, no such change occurs in the cells of the penis. The cells there are tough squamous cells and are resistant to attack. Penile cancer is very rare. Interestingly, though, HPV is implicated in around half the cases, and smoking has also emerged as a risk factor for this disease.

Can I prevent myself catching HPV?

As with any sexually transmitted infection, condoms will offer some protection. However, because HPV tends to spread invisibly all over the genital area, condoms do not guarantee safety. The diaphragm or cap is less likely to be effective, because there is even more genital contact. It would seem sensible to avoid smoking. The big problem, of course, is that you can't tell a man has HPV just by looking. Obviously, the more partners you have, the greater your chances of finding one who has HPV, but you could be unlucky and 'hit the jackpot' with the first.

Both men and women who are told they have HPV, or who develop visible genital warts, are often very upset at the inference that they must have been unfaithful, especially since they are often in a long-term monogamous relationship. However, the incubation period of the viruses can be very long, even years. So a virus you caught in a previous relationship may surface much later.

How infectious is HPV? Genital warts can certainly be passed on. But what about invisible HPV infection? Nobody actually knows. And if it is infectious, is that true all the time or just some of the time? And since you don't know you've got it, how can you know if you've got rid of it, or if you have passed it on? This is a very difficult area, and is one of the problems involved in testing for HPV (see below).

Treatment of HPV infections

Viruses are in fact very difficult to 'kill', since they are only susceptible when they are reproducing; often the only way to eliminate them is to kill the cells that are supporting them. If they have invaded a large number of cells, there is a danger that treatment aimed at eliminating the virus may kill the person as well.

So far, no treatment has been found that eradicates viruses completely and permanently. For example, a medicine called aciclovir is useful in the treatment of a herpes attack. It stops the replication of the herpes virus in infected cells, but leaves normal uninfected cells untouched. It therefore has very few side effects. Unfortunately, because it only affects cells in which the virus is replicating, it has no effect on cells where the virus is lying dormant, so these can surface and cause another attack.

Local treatments for visible warts all suffer the disadvantage that, obviously, they will only work where they are applied. As we have seen, HPV may be present in cells without causing visible warts; indeed, the more dangerous types (those associated with cancer) are precisely the ones that are 'invisible'. This does not mean, however, that visible genital warts should be ignored. They can become very large and unsightly.

It is difficult to say which treatment is best; one of the major problems is that genital warts often go away on their own, only to return later, so it can be difficult to tell whether it was, in fact, the treatment that made them go away. There are several chemicals that can be applied directly to genital warts. Podophyllotoxin (Condyline, Warticon) and imiquimod (Aldara) are prescribed for use at home. The other treatments, such as podophyllin, and trichloroacetic acid (TCA) are administered in clinics. Treatment can be time consuming, as the substance has to be applied regularly, often for several weeks, before the warts disappear. They can cause irritation and even burns if they are applied too heavily or too often. The treatments for abnormal cells (e.g. laser, cryotherapy, see Chapter 5) can be also used to treat warts, and may be faster, but they have not been shown to be more effective than chemical treatments in the long term.

Unfortunately, there is no treatment for invisible HPV infection caused by the 'high-risk' types. Clearly, it is not practical (or even safe, given the potential side effects) to just cover the entire genital area with chemicals. Research is ongoing, particularly looking at the use of imiquimod cream, which is already used for the treatment of visible warts: this works by boosting the local immune response, so it makes sense. However, the cervical skin is more delicate than that of the vulva, so it has proved more problematic to administer the cream without producing troublesome side effects.

You may ask, what is the point of treating women for CIN if they are going to return to an HPV-infected man? Won't they just get it back again? Interestingly, this does not often seem to be the case. It appears that when you remove the vulnerable area – the transformation zone – the risk of developing CIN again is actually quite small, around 10%. Thus, although these women may well still have HPV, and may be in a relationship with a man who has HPV, the virus cannot find vulnerable cells to invade and transform.

Testing for HPV

It seems obvious that, if HPV is the main cause of cervical cancer, we should be trying to detect it. Over the last 15 years, tests for HPV have evolved by leaps and bounds. A technique called polymerase chain reaction or PCR has enabled HPV types to be studied in great detail. PCR works rather like an enormous magnifying glass. Only a very tiny amount of the HPV DNA has to be present; the reagents have been primed to recognise a particular, specific variety of DNA. Once that is found, even in only one cell, it will be 'amplified', meaning that the reagents will take that piece of DNA, use it as a template and produce a huge number of copies. When enough copies are present, they become identifiable by special techniques and it is then possible to say that a particular virus type is there. This is a strength of PCR, that it can actually tell you the exact type or types of HPV present.

Before PCR, the techniques available were not as sensitive; therefore large amounts of the virus had to be present before it could be detected. Also the methods used were extremely slow and laborious. PCR is relatively quick and simple, and is extremely sensitive, being able to detect really minute amounts of virus. However, this very sensitivity can also cause problems. If you can pick up virus from just one cell, then if a few cells happen to be lying around on the workbench, and are wiped onto your test tube, your next experiment may apparently show HPV where it doesn't actually exist.

There is another new test for HPV, called Hybrid Capture (you may also see it referred to as HCII). This is set up to detect any of the 15 'high-risk' HPV types, without specifying which of them are present – you just get a positive or negative result. It is easier to perform and standardise than PCR, and for this reason has become the test that is widely used and commercially available. However, not being able to distinguish between the different HPV types is a disadvantage, because some types are more strongly associated with cancer than others.

Many studies have shown that HPV tests pick up cervical abnormalities that have been missed by cervical smears. But there is a problem, which comes back to the fact the HPV infection is so common and usually transient. You might have an HPV infection today, but by next month it may have gone. And just because there is an HPV infection at the moment, that doesn't mean it is doing any harm. HPV has to sit around in cells for years before it can cause CIN and cancer. Studies in which all women whose HPV tests are positive have a colposcopy, have shown that only around half of them have any abnormal cells (CIN). So for every women for whom the HPV test is useful, a second woman gets worried and has a colposcopy for no reason. Not to mention all the soul searching about where the infection came from – this is discussed in more detail in Chapter 10. It also has to be said that we cannot be absolutely sure, when there are no abnormal cells, that the HPV test was actually correct – maybe there wasn't HPV present at all, and it was a 'false positive'. No test is infallible.

However, what does seem to be true is that a negative HPV test is a good guarantee of safety. Since there are, effectively, no cancers without HPV, if you have a negative HPV test you can rest easy.

So how could HPV testing be used? It could be used as a screening test, like the smear. However, in young women (under 30), it would be pretty useless, because so many would have a positive test and be worried unnecessarily, simply because the infection is so common, transient and doing no harm. And then all the issues about whether it is infectious, the fact that there is no treatment, how you could know it had gone, these all surface and become a nightmare.

In older women (over 35) there may be a role, because fewer of them are likely to have a positive test, and, if they do, there is a greater likelihood that it is due to a persistent infection (i.e. one they caught some time back, but have not got rid of). That means that it is more likely there will be abnormal cells and so the test will have proved useful. But even in this group of women, many will have nothing wrong and will be worried for no reason.

It has been suggested that a single positive HPV test should not be acted upon, that women should wait 6 months or a year and have a repeat test. That way, if the infection were transient, it has been given time to clear, and they should only have a colposcopy if the repeat test is also positive. Sounds sensible, but I wonder how many people would be happy walking around for a year thinking about the fact that they have an HPV infection, not knowing if they are infectious, not being sure if there is anything more serious wrong. I think this is a very difficult issue and I don't have an answer, other than to say that knowledge usually empowers, so at least if women are aware of the issues, perhaps they will cope better. Unfortunately, as we shall see in Chapter 10, very few have this knowledge, which is one of the main reasons for this book.

HPV testing could be combined with cytology, so you could have an HPV test first, and only have a smear if it is positive. Liquid-based cytology (see Chapter 1) would allow all this to be done from the same sample, avoiding the need to have a second examination. Then, if the smear was abnormal, you would be referred for colposcopy. I don't know how reassured women would be if the smear was negative, though, because women are generally aware that smears can miss abnormalities. Again, there is no simple answer.

Another suggestion is not to use HPV testing for screening, but to use it in the management of women who have a borderline abnormal smear.

Borderline smears are a real problem nowadays: because smears rely on a subjective assessment by eye, cytologists tend to err on the side of caution (especially after the widely reported tragedies of women being missed). If there is any doubt, they will call it borderline, and of course, different people may have different opinions on the same slide, especially in the minor degrees of abnormality. So here we could utilise the reassurance that a negative HPV test can bring. Again, liquid cytology allows an HPV test to be performed on a smear sample without the woman having to return for another examination. So if she has a borderline smear, an HPV test could then be done; if it is negative, you can be pretty certain there is nothing to worry about, and those women needn't have colposcopy, or even 6-monthly smears. Of course, if the HPV test is positive, we are back to all the issues mentioned.

I think you can probably see by now that there is no perfect, or indeed simple, solution to this dilemma. While acknowledging this, we must not lose sight of the fact that the screening programme has been very successful in the UK (see Chapter 9), and currently you are best advised to have regular smears.

The ultimate solution, which is now on the horizon, is prevention of cervical cancer with a vaccine against HPV. This is discussed in Chapter 11.

9 THE CERVICAL SCREENING CONTROVERSY: HOW OFTEN SHOULD YOU HAVE A SMEAR?

The first question is: why bother to have smears at all? It's not as stupid as it sounds. Screening is only worthwhile if certain things are true about the disease you are looking for. It must be reasonably common, or a lot of people will go through the bother of having the test when there is virtually no chance of them having the condition. The test used should be simple and accurate: people should not be frightened unnecessarily, nor be given false reassurance. The disease you are looking for must be curable; there is no point finding it just to tell people they are going to die. Ideally, the test should be able to detect the disease so early that complete cure is possible in every case.

Cervical cancer is unusual amongst cancers in that it has an 'early warning' stage, CIN, which is present for several years before actual cancer develops. This makes it a perfect candidate for screening as, theoretically, we should be able to pick up most abnormalities before they have turned into cancer.

Why should I go for a test? I feel perfectly OK.

Isn't it something you only get if you sleep around? I don't want my neighbours seeing me at the doctor's – they might get the wrong idea.

Currently, in the UK, around 3000 women a year develop cervical cancer. Many of those women have never had a smear. They do not go for tests for a variety of reasons. Some feel that they will be thought promiscuous because they have heard that the disease is related to promiscuity. Older people are less used to the concept of screening; they only go to see the doctor when they are ill. Many women think the smear is a test for cancer itself, rather than for 'early warning' changes – and they would rather not know if they have cancer. All these misunderstandings arise from a lack of information, about what

115

the smear is, what the possible causes of cervical cancer are, how CIN can be treated and how effective the treatment is. Ignorance breeds fear and women who are frightened of having a smear are very unlikely to go for one. Unfortunately, such women are also unlikely to be reading a book like this: maybe you have a friend who has never had a smear and is frightened; please pass on what you have learned to her.

As you can see from Figure 9.1, cervical cancer rates start to rise after the age of 25 and are at their highest between the ages of 30 and 45.

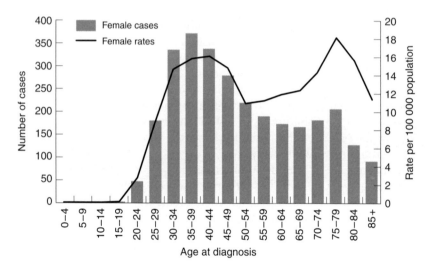

Figure 9.1 Cervical cancer incidence rate per 100 000, UK, 2001. Reproduced from the Cancer Research UK website: http://info.cancerresearchuk.org/cancerstats/types/cervix/incidence/

Young women have been the group in whom cervical cancer rates have been increasing most rapidly. It is often said that too many smears are taken from young women, who are supposedly at low risk. And yet this increase in women under 35 has occurred despite the fact that they are having 'too many' smears. One can only speculate as to what the figures would have been if they had not had them.

You will notice in Figure 9.2 that the incidence (i.e. the number of cases) of cervical cancer has been going down since about 1990. It is no

116

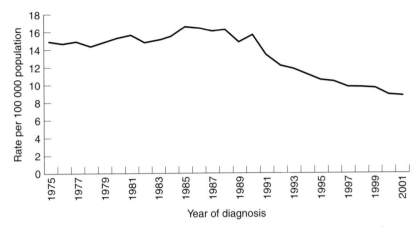

Figure 9.2 Trends in age standardised incidence rates per 100 000 population for cervical cancer, 1975–2001, Great Britain. Reproduced from the Cancer Research UK website: http://info.cancerresearchuk.org/cancerstats/types/cervix/incidence/

coincidence that the NHS Cervical Screening Programme started to be fully functional in about 1988. It has been a great success story, despite the media scare stories which appear at regular intervals.

How often should I have a smear?

It's quite simple, actually – the more frequently you have them the better your protection will be. And so to move on to the next section … .

Yes it really is that simple. These calculations have been done many times and the answer is always the same. So why is there so much argument about the frequency of smears? You guessed it – money.

There is another aspect, of course. How often would you like to go for a smear? Every 5 years? Every 3 years? Every year? Perhaps you're really worried and you'd like to go every 6 months – why stop at that, get to know your doctor really well, go every week … you can see that this could become quite ridiculous. I have yet to meet a woman who actually enjoys having a smear (no letters please!). There has to be a point at which you get no extra protection for your discomfort. Also, as mentioned in Chapter 2, some women will be made more anxious, perhaps unnecessarily so, by a mildly abnormal smear. Some may receive

Table 9.1 Relative protection against cervical cancer according to frequency of smear tests

Months since last negative smear	Relative protection
0–11	15.3
12–23	11.9
24–35	8.0
36–47	5.3
48–59	2.8
Never screened	1.0

Data from IARC. *BMJ* 1986; **293**: 659–664.

treatment they did not really need; the likelihood of all this increases with the frequency at which you have smears.

Table 9.1 is taken from several large international studies, whose results were pooled and published in 1986 – many different studies have been done, the exact numbers vary, but the principle remains the same. The woman who has never been screened is assumed to be the standard, with a risk of 1.0. The woman who has yearly or 2-yearly smears is 12 times less likely to develop cancer. However, the woman who has five yearly smears is only three times less likely to develop cancer. It follows therefore that yearly/2-yearly screening is more effective at protecting against cervical cancer than is 5-yearly screening. Put another way, annual smears could possibly prevent 92% of cervical cancer, whereas 5-yearly screening could prevent 67%.

There is a contradiction here: if cervical cancer takes around 10 years to develop, surely 5-yearly screening would be enough? And yet the figures show clearly that it isn't. The problem lies with the smear test itself; smears can be wrong, and give false reassurance. In fact, for the lower grades of CIN, the false-negative rate (by which I mean that an abnormality was present, but the smear missed it) can be as high as 50%. Before you go into a panic, let me stress that this does not mean that half the smears taken give the wrong result. What it does mean is that the smear may be missing up to half the cases of mild abnormality. Only about 5–10% of women who have smears have a mild abnormality, so only about 5–10% of women are actually getting a false-negative result.

Why do smears give the wrong result? There seem to be three reasons. First, the smear may not be taken in the right way or from the right place.

There have been several reports where doctors or nurses have been found to be using tongue depressors, for example, to take smears. In another case, a speculum was not being used, so the cervix was not seen. Obviously, whatever instrument is being used, if it is not wiped across the cervix, the result will have no meaning. Similarly, even when the cervix can be seen, part of it may be missed when taking the smear: that might be just the area that was abnormal. Chapters 1 and 3 discussed the use of newer instruments that have been designed to try and make smears more accurate. In Chapter 3, I also mentioned the debate about the importance, or otherwise, of endocervical cells. These issues have still not been resolved. Some studies suggest that endocervical cells are important, others say they are not. The bottom line is probably that the person taking the smear is more important than the instrument being used: if you have someone who is good at taking smears, they will probably take a good smear with any (reasonable) instrument you give them. One of the problems with such studies is that the chances are that the doctors and nurses who volunteer to take part may be precisely the interested and experienced ones who will do well anyway. This is likely to make it more difficult to tell whether one instrument would be better than another in less experienced hands.

When you go for a smear, you yourself can make a difference to the outcome, If you are tense, it can be very difficult to see your cervix: the doctor or nurse may do their best, but in the end it is you who suffers if the smear was not taken well.

Mistakes can occur in the cytology laboratory. Spare a thought for rows of cytology screeners, who have to look down microscopes all day, every day. The vast majority of slides they see – around 90% – will be normal, so their work is unbelievably monotonous. Is it any wonder their concentration can lapse occasionally? Indeed, it has been shown that slides looked at on Monday morning or Friday afternoon are more likely to be misinterpreted. For this reason, systems have been set up in laboratories to double-check the process, so that any errors are spotted quickly.

Some smears (around 8%) may be called negative when they are actually not good enough for interpretation, perhaps because there is too much blood obscuring the cells. Again, hopefully these may be picked up by a second check, and this particular problem will be reduced by the introduction of liquid-based cytology (see Chapter 2)

There is another worrying aspect of the misinterpretation of slides. It has been shown that if two different cytologists look at the same

119

slide, they are quite likely to grade it differently. Not only that, but the same cytologist may give a different opinion on the same slide on different days. The majority of such differences occur in the 'grey areas', rather than the barn-door severely abnormal smears. Nevertheless, the consequences can be serious if a woman whose smear actually shows an abnormality is given the all clear and advised to have her next smear in 5 years. It would obviously be better all round if the 'human error' aspect of cytology could somehow be removed.

The last reason why smears can be falsely negative is the most puzzling. It seems that while one cervix sheds cells easily, another does not. Maybe a cervix with only a mild abnormality is less likely to shed cells than one that has a more severe abnormality. This is not unreasonable, since, as we saw in Chapter 2, there will be a greater thickness of cells involved the higher the degree of abnormality, so it should be easier to dislodge a few. However, it is known that a cervix that has already developed actual cancer may also give a negative smear. This aspect is probably beyond our control.

The bottom line is that single smear results, taken in isolation, are not always reliable. However, it is very unlikely that a succession of negative smears taken from the same woman will all be false negatives. This is the explanation of the paradox we encountered earlier: cervical cancer takes around 10 years to develop, but relatively frequent smears are required to give the maximum protection against it. If a woman is having yearly smears, an occasional false-negative result does not matter: she will have an accurate result within a year or two, which should be well in time to show up an abnormality before it becomes a cancer. However, if the same woman is only having a smear once every 5 years, the situation is quite different. If she has a false-negative smear, there is then a 10-year gap between her last real negative smear and the date her next smear is due. This is too long and she may then find that she does have cancer, despite having had a 'negative' smear within the last 5 years.

OK, so why does the government tell you that you can only have a smear every 3 or 5 years? Because it is being advised by people who consider the global view. It is quite definitely true that in countries like Finland, where screening is done only once every 5 years, there has been a considerable reduction in the incidence of cervical cancer (see Table 9.2).

120

Table 9.2 Percentage reduction in cumulative risk of cervical cancer in the age range 35–64, with different screening histories

Screening frequency (years)	Reduction in risk (%)	Number of tests (35–64 age range)
1	93.3	30
2	93.3	15
3	91.4	10
5	83.9	6
10	64.2	3

Adapted from IARC. *BMJ* 1986; **293**: 659–664.

Table 9.2 shows you that screening every 3 years, on a national level, gives almost the same level of protection as screening every year (a 91% reduction in risk as opposed to a 93% reduction). Even 5-yearly screening gives an 83% reduction in risk. But look again at the last column in the table, which shows how many smears each woman would have to have. If your screening programme works on a 3-yearly basis, you only need 10 smears per woman, as opposed to 30 if they were done yearly – one-third of the number. And you only get an extra 2% reduction in risk for your 20 extra smears per woman. Financially, I think you have to admit, it makes sense for a country to run a 3-yearly screening programme. In fact, there are those who will argue that 5-yearly screening makes just about as much sense, but the general consensus in the medical profession has been to advise 3-yearly screening programmes.

Screening programmes are very, very costly to run and financial decisions have to be made. A yearly screening programme would be ruinously expensive and really wouldn't save many extra lives compared to a 3-yearly programme. Indeed, if you look again at Table 9.2, you'll see that there is no difference between yearly and 2-yearly screening, so actually annual smears are probably a waste of time and money. Although in many countries women are advised to have yearly smears, they nearly always have to pay for those smears themselves, or have them done through insurance schemes. I cannot think of any country that runs a free yearly screening programme. It therefore seems to me that at present we cannot expect the government to fund a screening programme running on more than a 3-yearly basis.

There are groups of women who need more frequent screening anyway, and who obtain this within the screening programme, for example women who have already had an abnormal smear, or those who have been treated for CIN.

Another vexed question is: when should women start having smears? This debate is currently raging in the UK, because the starting age was recently raised from 20 to 25. The reasoning goes like this: invasive cervical cancer is very rare in women under 25. In 2002, 26 cases of invasive cervical cancer were registered for women aged between 15 and 24. Indeed, it has been suggested that screening women under the age of 25 may do more harm than good. Young women frequently have borderline or mildly abnormal smears and yet, when referred for colposcopy, are not found to have any disease. Such false-positive results lead to a lot of unnecessary investigation and anxiety. Even worse, they can lead to unnecessary treatments, which may scar them psychologically (see Chapter 10). This is all true. However, many doctors are worried about the change because they point out that the calculations used did not include microinvasive disease, which is not so rare in young women. Although they do not die, having a hysterectomy in your twenties is likely to have a devastating effect psychologically, removing the chances of having children and having to come to terms with all that involves. In addition, they point out that sexual behaviour has been changing over the last 10–15 years, and because cervical cancer takes 10 years to develop, inevitably statistics lag behind. We know that early age at first sexual intercourse is a risk factor for cervical cancer, and the proportion of women who start having sex earlier is increasing all the time. Surveys show that the age at first intercourse has been steadily falling, from an average of 21 years for women born in the 1930s, to 17 years for those born in the 1960s. And the proportion having their first intercourse under the age of 16 has been increasing, from 1% in those born in the 1930s to 25% in those born in the late 1970s (these figures come from the National Sexual Attitudes and Lifestyles Surveys, 1994 and 2001).

In many countries, the age at commencement of screening is linked to the start of sexual activity, which is logical in some ways. However, I do think we have to balance the benefits against the risks. Although women are having sex earlier, and a lot of abnormal smears do get picked up in teenagers, it really is true that there is virtually no cervical cancer, invasive or microinvasive, under the age of 20. So I think screening teenagers, subjecting them to embarrassing examinations and unnecessary colposcopies and treatments, is going too far. Nevertheless, like many doctors, I am concerned at the recent rise in starting age to 25 years, and hope

122

that careful monitoring will be taking place, so that, if the policy is shown to be less safe, it can be changed back quickly. Only time will tell.

At the same time as the change in starting age, there has been a change in the frequency of screening at different ages. Whereas previously, the screening programme recommended 5-yearly screening as a minimum, and 3-yearly screening as optional, now women between 25 and 49 will have 3-yearly screening, while those between 50 and 64 will have 5-yearly screening. This is based on the fact that, as shown in Figure 9.1, women between 30 and 45 are at highest risk.

So what should you, as a woman, do about having smears? First of all, make sure you are getting your share of the screening programme: respond to the reminder. Some women think they can only have their smear with their GP, and are embarrassed to do so, especially if he is male and has known them since childhood. But in fact, you are entitled to have your screening smear with other doctors: your GP may have a female partner or a nurse, who could do your smear. If that is not the case, you can actually go to another GP, with whom you are not registered, just for a smear. Or you can go to a family planning or well woman clinic. Family planning clinics do not usually require a letter from your GP before they will do a smear, you can just make your own appointment. However, one problem with the current system is that you must be registered with a GP in order to have a smear. This is because the GP is the person deemed responsible for making sure you get your results and any referral or follow-up if necessary. This can be a real problem for young women in cities, where the GP lists are often full, and they move frequently anyway. I've seen women who really want to have a smear taken, and who are overdue for one, but can't get it done at a family planning clinic simply because they are not registered with a GP. Both they and I find this frustrating and ridiculous.

What if you want to have more frequent smears? Still go for your NHS smear – why not take up a free offer? You can always then pay for a smear in between, if you want to. Private clinics will do a smear for around £50, including the consultation fee. But if this is too much, remember that the screening programme is still giving you a good level of protection. I expect some readers will be angry that I can even suggest women might pay for some of their smears. But life is not fair and no government will fund more than 3-yearly screening – I have shown you why. So I am simply saying what you might do if you want a higher level of protection than the screening programme can give.

When can I stop having smears?

The current government guidelines are that women should have smears until the age of 64. This seems quite reasonable: as we have seen, in fact CIN is more common in younger women, so provided you have had regular smears up till then, it is not very likely that you will develop cervical cancer after you have retired. Although women over 65 do get cervical cancer, the vast majority have never had a smear, or had not had adequate screening.

Some doctors have suggested that women over 50, who have previously had normal smears, could stop at that age, rather than 64. I would caution against this view. It seems to be traditionally thought that women over 50 are at lower risk of getting cervical cancer – after all, who is up to anything at that age anyway? But, of course, if we look at what is going on in society at the moment, we can see that it is at precisely that time of life that divorces are becoming increasingly common. As a result, people form new relationships and, with new partners come new risks of infection. Several studies have now recorded a recent rise in sexually transmitted infection rates (including HPV) in people in their forties and fifties. I worry that in 10 years' time, the same will be seen to be happening to rates of cervical cancer.

There have also been suggestions that women should have tests even later in life. This is certainly true if you have never had a smear, or have not had one for a long time. However, if you have had regular smears and they have been negative, I feel the disadvantages outweigh the advantages. Having smears in your late sixties and seventies is often increasingly uncomfortable, especially if you are not taking hormone replacement therapy. The vagina becomes less elastic, so opening the speculum is more difficult and can be very painful. In addition, the smears can be more difficult to interpret, because as the cells lose oestrogen (a hormone), they shrink and tend to look a little like abnormal cells.

What if you have had a hysterectomy (removal of the uterus, or womb)? If the operation was performed for a problem unrelated to cervical cancer (e.g. heavy periods, fibroids), you need not have further smears, regardless of your age. However, if the hysterectomy was done because of cervical cancer, you should have yearly vaginal smears for at least the next 10 years, and probably for longer.

Making sure you get your smear result

Having gone to all the effort of having a smear done, it must be worth making sure you know what the result is. And yet women often forget when and where they last had a smear. Sometimes they have had a smear during a gynaecological check-up but are unaware it was done. This may lead to unnecessary duplication of smears, but may also result in a situation where smears are assumed to have been taken when in fact they were not. Some clinics and GPs give women a personalised 'cervical smear record card' so that she can record the date and result of her last smear. Even if they don't, it is not such a big effort to create such a page in your diary.

You may have read about women who, for one reason or another, did not receive their smear results: because of this, they did not have follow-up checks and subsequently died of cancer. Mistakes are always going to happen. Nowadays, you are supposed to be informed of your result, even if it is negative. However, this system will break down if you are not registered with a GP, if you move, or if it just gets lost in the post. In the end, it is up to you to make sure you know when you last had a smear and to find out the result. After all, it is your life that may be at risk. It is a mistake to rely on other people to take this responsibility. They may be dealing with thousands of results; you are only interested in one, your own. Who is the more likely to lose it?

Having read this book, you should be in a position to understand what your smear result means. There is nothing to stop you asking to see the report for yourself. Don't get fobbed off by doctors or nurses who tell you it might frighten you: that's why you have devoted the time to finding out what the form means. And if there is something on it that you don't understand, well, they will just have to explain it. That is what they are there for.

I'm not saying you should be on the phone to your doctor within a week of having a smear. Ask how long the results usually take, allow a couple of weeks' grace for inefficiency, postal delays and so on and make a note in your diary of when to check if you have not been notified. Sometimes it is helpful to leave a stamped addressed envelope in your records. Or, if you know you are coming back for an appointment anyway in the next few months, check then. Even if you leave it till your next 6-monthly family planning appointment – which is likely to be perfectly safe – ask, in case the result has been filed and forgotten, or never came back from the lab.

In 1999, I went for a routine smear. My life was very busy, I was working hard, travelling a lot. I guess I forgot about the smear really, I just assumed that since I hadn't heard it must be OK. A year later I had some discharge and went to the doctor, a different one as I had moved again. She didn't have my records yet, so she did a smear anyway, since I couldn't remember exactly how long it was since I'd had one. A month later I was posted to the States for a year. In the excitement, I forgot to let the clinic know – well, you tell your friends and your family, but you can't remember everything. When I came back from the States, I was a bit worried as I'd had some funny bleeding every now and again. I hadn't wanted to see anyone in the States: it was expensive and I thought there was no point since I'd be back home soon. I found a flat in the same area as before, so I went to the doctor I'd seen for the last smear. She was frantic. Hadn't I got the letter a year ago? It turned out that not only the smear she had done, but the one before that were both abnormal. She referred me to the hospital straight away, but it was too late. I had cancer. I had to have a hysterectomy and radiotherapy afterwards. I was 34 then, now I'm 36. It's taken me a long time to come to terms with it, I'm not sure I have yet. People my age don't get cancer. It's not fair.

I have embellished the details a little, but this was a true story. Don't let it be yours.

10 EMOTIONAL FEELINGS AND REACTIONS

One of the prerequisites of screening is that the process should not cause psychological harm to those involved. For a long time, this aspect was ignored with regard to cervical screening: after all, here was a test which could actually *prevent* women developing cancer, it was one of the most wonderful advances in medicine. It was unthinkable that it could cause harm; surely women would be overjoyed at this protection they were getting?

However, it has been increasingly realised that women do in fact suffer emotionally as a result of the whole screening and treatment process. Where previously research concentrated on purely physical aspects, in recent years a number of studies have been carried out to look at the psychological effects of screening, colposcopy and treatment. You will find details of a couple of books written specifically on this subject in the Further Reading section.

The one thing that emerges as the most important cause of anxiety is lack of information and understanding as to why smears are taken and what it means if they are abnormal. This is not a new concept: 'ignorance breeds fear' is an old saying. The other big problems are the embarrassment of the procedures involved and the association of cervical cancer with sexual behaviour.

Deciding to have a smear

Yes, I meant to have a smear test. I kept meaning to go. But I always had a reason I couldn't: I was too busy, it was the wrong time of the month, I wasn't feeling up to it.

The thought of the examination put me off. So undignified, I couldn't have such a thing done by a man.

Even the decision to go for a smear is not an easy one. The examination is embarrassing and many women do not realise that they can insist on seeing a female doctor, even at another practice or clinic, for a smear.

Why should I have a smear? There's nothing wrong with me. I'll just be wasting the doctor's time.

It's a test for cancer, isn't it? Well. I'd rather not know – once you get cancer you're dead.

The commonest misconception is that smears test for cancer, which, as we have seen, is just not true. The whole point of smears is to pick up changes in cells, CIN, which are not cancer and which can be completely removed before they ever get the chance to become cancer.

Again, women think that they don't need tests because they are well. But the idea is to detect CIN before it ever becomes so serious as to turn into cancer and produce symptoms. Indeed, women are often worried when they have a discharge or bleeding, but actually there is only a small chance that these problems will turn out to be related to cervical cancer or CIN. A discharge is much more likely to be caused by infection. Bleeding after sex can be a sign of cervical cancer, but is much more commonly caused by a cervical ectropion or erosion (see Chapter 3).

Why should I have a smear? I've only slept with one man, my husband.

As we have seen, although there is an association between women's sexual behaviour and cervical cancer, the behaviour of the man is equally important. So, although a woman may have been faithful, her partner may place her at risk. It is also important to remember that there are other factors involved, not just sexual behaviour. We know that smoking is likely to be involved, that the immune system is important, but there are still plenty of things we do not know. Sexual behaviour is not the only factor, there may be something else, something we have not suspected, which plays a vital part.

I'm too old. I haven't had sex for years and years.

Age is unimportant, nor when you last had sex. If you have not had regular smears, you should still have one, even if you are 70. Many women think that once they have passed through the menopause (change of life), the womb no longer has a function and nothing else will happen 'down there' either. This is not true.

The smear test itself

It is unfortunate if, having psyched yourself up to have a smear, the examination turns out to be unpleasant. Not only is this traumatic at the time, but it will sour your attitude to future tests, maybe put you off altogether. Most women find that the examination is actually not as bad as they expected and are relieved to find how quick and simple it was. You can do quite a lot to help yourself, by trying to be as relaxed as possible both before and during the examination. Don't choose to have your smear on the same day as a stressful meeting at work, bring a friend along if you think it will help. Do some relaxation exercises, have a stiff drink, some women get themselves into such a state they need tranquillisers.

If they have not already done so, ask the doctor or nurse to warm the speculum, for example under the hot tap. A freezing cold metal instrument is no fun at all. If there is an observer in the room, for example a student, remember that you are at liberty to ask for them to leave. They need to learn, but if you are very tense, your needs come first. It is likely that there will be a curtain round the couch, but if there is not (and even if there is, if it will make you feel better) ask for the door to be locked. Having a smear only takes a minute, but if you are worried about someone coming in, even a nurse, it will make the process more difficult.

If there is a reason why you are particularly nervous (for example a bad previous experience, a sexual assault in the past), mention it at the start. Although everyone is (hopefully) treated with care, it will alert the doctor or nurse to take more time and be aware that the examination may be difficult.

Once you have had the smear, make sure you find out what the result was. The importance of this is discussed in Chapter 9.

An abnormal, 'positive' smear result

You are a perfectly rational woman. You have a responsible position, a career, a family to look after. Normally you are a rock. You receive a letter which says 'your cervical smear test showed an abnormality. Please make an appointment to discuss this at your earliest convenience'. In an instant you turn into a gibbering wreck.

> I just thought: 'I'm going to die.' I went numb, I couldn't move. I stood there holding the letter and crying.

Yes, I went regularly for smears, but I never thought I'd have anything wrong. I thought the smear protected you.

I made the mistake of phoning my mother. She made it worse, she started to cry on the phone, saying she couldn't believe she was going to lose her only daughter.

Why me, what did I do?

A reaction combining shock, disbelief, guilt and anger is very common. Some women remain calm, but they are in a minority. The reaction is mostly due to the fear of cancer, even in women who, under normal circumstances, know that an abnormal smear does not mean cancer. Even nurses and doctors, who are well informed, can be frightened, deep down.

I was devastated. Robert and I had been together for 4 years and we had just told our parents we were going to get married and start a family. My first thought was that I'd never have children.

As we have seen, the treatments for CIN do not affect your fertility. However, many women do not realise this and it is a major source of anxiety.

After the initial shock, I started thinking: 'why did it happen to me? I haven't been promiscuous. What will John say? What will he think?' I remembered I'd had a fling just once during our marriage. It was only one night, after a dinner, when I was away on a course. I'd never mentioned it to John. I felt terrible. Maybe it was all my fault, maybe this was my punishment.'

Some women blame themselves, others turn on their partner. Did he pass on HPV, is he the one to blame? This, in turn may make him feel guilty and rejected. Relationships can suffer at this time because of accusations in both directions and most likely all unnecessary.

A supportive partner can be a great help at this time: remember that the chances are he is worried, even if he is not showing it. Many men do feel guilty, even without being reminded. Newspapers and magazines have spread the word about the 'high-risk male' quite widely. Men are often seen in sexually transmitted disease clinics asking to be checked for warts in case they might infect their girlfriends or wives. It is very frustrating for them to be told that there is no way they can be given an unconditional all clear – there is always the possibility of microscopic infection, for which nothing can be done. Unfortunately, some men go along looking for confirmation that they have no visible warts; if this is given, without the caution that there might be microscopic infection, they may go home and accuse their partner of being unfaithful, or tell her it must be her fault. Accusations from either partner are only hurtful and achieve nothing positive. It is far more useful for both partners to realise each other's fears and guilt and help each other through the experience.

The most important thing to do if you are informed of an abnormal smear is to discuss it fully with your doctor. Some doctors are better informed than others: hopefully yours will be able to give you the information you need. Otherwise, read as much as you can find on the subject. Talk to other women who have been through the experience already – only remember that their result may not have been the same as yours, so not everything may be applicable to you.

It is worth mentioning that some women and their partners are worried whether continuing to have sex might make the abnormal cells get worse. This is not the case: indeed, one could argue that you should make the most of your time, because if you have to have treatment, you will be advised to abstain for a month afterwards!

An inadequate smear

The letter just said the smear needed to be repeated because it didn't contain enough material. It said not to worry. But wouldn't they say that if they wanted to repeat it 'cause they weren't sure?

I knew it was just a routine repeat. But I couldn't stop thinking about it until I got the next result, telling me it was OK.

Unfortunately, many women think, when they are asked to have a repeat smear because the first one was inadequate, that we are trying to hide something. A study has shown that women receiving such a result are just as anxious as if they had been told they had an abnormal smear. Fortunately, the introduction of liquid-based cytology should greatly reduce the number of inadequate smears, and if it does nothing else, it will have been worth it. All I can say is, an inadequate smear result really does just mean it wasn't a good enough sample to report on – but I'm afraid, no matter how often I say it, deep down, you won't believe me.

Finding out you have HPV

Women generally know little about cervical smears, but they know even less about HPV. Most people have not even heard of HPV, let alone any link between it and cervical cancer. And even if they are aware that cervical cancer is in some way related to sexual activity, they don't link that to HPV. A large survey carried out recently in the UK found that only 1% of people had heard of HPV in relation to cervical cancer.

So where did this virus come from? How long could I have had it? Did my partner give to me? Has he been unfaithful?

These are questions I have heard (often through tears) again and again. Women are actually even more anxious about having HPV than about having an abnormal smear. A study has recently looked at the impact of the addition of an HPV test result for women who had a mild or borderline abnormal smear. They found that the women who were told they had a positive HPV test were more anxious than those who just had an abnormal smear. What was very sad was that women who had an abnormal smear, but were told their HPV test was negative, were just as anxious as if they had not had the test – and this is one situation in which an HPV test should be reassuring, as mentioned in Chapter 7. Once again, what came out strongly was that women simply didn't understand about HPV.

As I mentioned in Chapter 8, HPV infection is so common that it has been described as 'a natural consequence of having sex'. We have a 75% chance of catching it at some point, but in the vast majority of cases it will just go away on its own, like a cold. If only people knew that, and not only knew it, but *believed* it. This is the problem with HPV testing, that there is a high chance (particularly in young women) that the result will be positive, but there will be no abnormal cells there. Also, we have no way of knowing how long the virus has been around: weeks, months, even years. Both men and women can carry HPV for years without knowing. And when a woman has a negative smear, but a positive HPV test, anxiety and bewilderment mix together. The smear result does nothing to allay the fear.

I feel dirty, it's a sexually transmitted disease. Can I pass it on? How do I get rid of it? What can I do?

He says it must be me, he says he's never had warts. He called me a slag.

I was a virgin, I've never been with another man. I know he's been with other women. But he said it was my fault.

The worst thing about HPV is that there is no treatment. You can't see it's there, so you don't know how long it's been there, or when it's gone – if it's gone. Women have to live with that uncertainty. And the fact that genital warts are related to, though not the same as, the HPV types that cause abnormal smears, makes it even worse. Misunderstandings, such as those in the quotes above, cause enormous distress.

I typed 'HPV' into Google and there were pages and pages of sites. I looked at a few, but they didn't seem to say the same things, some said this, some said that, some talked about treating warts, it was all so confusing.

I tried to ask the doctor how long I might have had it, but he just said it wasn't worth worrying about things like that. We should just move on. But how will I ever know if it's gone away?

It is a problem that there is no control over what goes on the internet, so you can't be sure that what you read is correct. Or explained clearly. Or up to date. Research and understanding in this area has been moving so fast that there are lots of out-of-date sites out there. I have tried to list some reliable sources of information at the end of this book. Another problem is that we just don't have definitive answers to many of the questions. Many doctors and nurses find it hard to admit that they don't know the answers, especially if they are not too sure their own knowledge is up to date. You have to be pretty confident of your knowledge to be able to say 'there is no answer to that question' without fear of being proved wrong. So they may try not to answer, or to give a vague answer. Unfortunately, that may just result in more confusion.

In recent years researchers have started looking at people's understanding of the issues around HPV infection. What has come out most strongly is the need for more information and education about the link between HPV and cervical cancer. Since HPV testing may well become more common (see Chapter 8), and HPV vaccines are not far away (see Chapter 11), it is critical that people become better informed. Otherwise we have the potential to do more harm than good.

At the colposcopy clinic

In theory, if women attending colposcopy clinics were fully informed about the meaning of their smear results, they should not be anxious. However, even informed women often experience anxiety at the thought of the examination and what might be found.

Many women find the wait between the smear result and a colposcopy very stressful, especially if it takes several months (as often happens if you have only a mildly abnormal smear). It is always worth asking your GP if another hospital has a shorter waiting list – but check why: maybe it has a bad reputation! You can use the time constructively. Find out as much as you can about the procedure, the possible treatments, particularly what is likely to be on offer at the hospital you are going to attend. Check whether you are likely to be offered treatment on the same day as your initial examination, so called 'see and treat' clinics. These are discussed in detail in Chapter 4. The main practical implication for you is that you may need to make extra arrangements at home and work if you have treatment that day. Nowadays there are support groups in some areas, run by women who have gone through the experience of an abnormal smear. See if there is a local one you could go to.

If you are a smoker, maybe this could provide that final incentive to give up. However, do bear in mind that it is likely to be an additional cause of stress at a time when you are already tense and worried.

During the weeks before my appointment, I read all the books and leaflets I could get hold of. I went onto the internet and looked at loads of sites. Some of them contradicted each other, which was confusing. As I went along, I wrote down questions about things I didn't understand, or which didn't seem to be answered. Then, before I went to the hospital, I made a list of the questions I felt I should ask. Normally, I find I clam up when I'm faced with a doctor in a white coat. Having a list made it a lot easier.

Many doctors actually find it easier to answer questions than to think of things to say on their own, so don't be afraid to ask. Some questions may need to wait until after the examination, as the doctor will not know what is actually wrong with you until then.

The position you have to lie in during the colposcopy examination can be described, at best, as inelegant. Once again, relaxation is important, especially as the procedure will take longer than a smear. Do not hesitate to ask for privacy (for example by having the door locked): in some clinics doctors and nurses just wander in and out of the rooms without warning. They may be used to women lying with their legs in the air but you are not: they know who they are, but as far as you are concerned, they could be John Smith from the newspaper shop. The same applies to observers: they should be introduced to you first, and your permission requested for them to stay.

It is sometimes said that once you have had a baby you can never be embarrassed again. This is not true. For a start, having a baby is (one hopes) an experience that is expected to have a pleasant and rewarding outcome. Women therefore approach it in quite a different manner and perceive it differently. In addition, they are often so tired and so glad to get it over that they have ceased to care about elegance and privacy. Lastly, the memory of the actual labour and delivery, like many painful and unpleasant experiences, fades, and therefore cannot be readily drawn on for comparison. So do not let yourself be made to feel inadequate by this kind of statement, even though it may be well meant.

> I was so nervous before – and during the examination, for that matter. But afterwards, I was so relieved. At least I knew what was going on and that it wasn't cancer.

Most women feel much happier after their colposcopy, because the uncertainty has been removed. Make sure before you leave that you have asked all the questions you wanted to. It often helps to have your partner or a friend present because you may not be able to remember everything. I have often found myself repeating things several times within one consultation, because it is obvious that my patient has not taken in what I have said. It has occasionally been suggested that such conversations are taped, to be listened to again later, but I think some doctors would find that daunting and you might find that they were less open and helpful – not necessarily consciously, but just through 'stage fright'.

If you have not seen it in a book or a leaflet, take the opportunity to get the doctor to draw you a picture of your cervix, or show you a photograph, if that is possible. Many women seem to have the idea that the abnormal area is somehow mouldy, or fungating, or a black hole. It makes everything much less frightening if you know what it really looks like. Some clinics have the colposcope wired up to a TV monitor, so you can see what is going on: again, although some women find this really interesting and useful, others find it scary. If you don't want to see, just say so.

Unfortunately, the colposcopy is usually followed by another period of waiting and anxiety, before the biopsy result comes back. (Indeed, you may also have to wait for the result of another smear, which usually takes longer.) You may be given another appointment for this, or, more often, you will be informed by letter. This is why it is so important that you have thought through and discussed all the options by the end of your colposcopy visit; you may not easily have another chance to talk to the specialist until your treatment or next colposcopy appointment. If you do find you have been taken by surprise, do not be frightened to ask for another appointment to discuss it again. It is very unlikely you would be refused; most doctors working in this field know how anxious women become and will be sympathetic.

Treatment

Although some clinics now treat women at the same visit as the initial colposcopy, it is more common to have the treatment performed at a separate visit. You may see this as an advantage, a chance to prepare yourself and learn more about the problem. However, the waiting can make some women very anxious. Relationships with families and friends suffer because you are tense and irritable, your performance at work declines and so on. Do not struggle on by yourself; counselling may help.

Most women find that they are pleasantly surprised and relieved once they have had their treatment. It is not nearly as painful or traumatic as they expected. However, the thought that part of their cervix has had to be destroyed leaves some women with psychological and psychosexual problems. A study has been done, which compared women who had abnormal smears with those who had come into contact with a sexually transmitted disease, non-specific urethritis (or chlamydia). The study looked at features such as interest in sex, feelings towards the partner, pain during sex and satisfaction with sex. Women who had an abnormal smear necessitating colposcopy and treatment were found to have far more negative feelings towards sex than those who knew their partners had non-specific urethritis and were treated for it themselves.

It is also interesting that it did not seem to be the abnormal smear itself which was associated with psychosexual problems. No change in attitude was noted from the time the women knew their smear was abnormal to the time they had their colposcopy, even though, in many cases, this interval amounted to several months. However, their attitudes changed significantly *after* they had had colposcopy and treatment. They showed loss of interest in sex, felt hostile towards their partner, did not enjoy sex as much as before, and often said they experienced pain during intercourse.

Of course, these feelings are often related to one another, and may be related most of all to the woman's anxiety. For example, a woman who is feeling anxious about her cervix may well be worried about having sex. She is therefore not very relaxed during intercourse and does not find the experience as pleasant and satisfying as before. Anxiety about her sexual performance may then be added to her other worries. Her partner may feel rejected and the relationship may suffer. When she has sex again, she will be even more anxious than before, will thus be more tense, find it more uncomfortable and the experience will be even less pleasant for both partners. A vicious circle soon develops, as a result of which she is likely to feel that it is preferable not to have sex at all and avoid the issue altogether.

> I found it really hard to have sex. On one hand, I was frightened of losing Richard and adding to my problems. On the other, the last thing I was interested in was doing something which constantly reminded me of the abnormality.

The results of this study are worrying. More and more young women are developing CIN; they may not yet have found a stable relationship or started their family. It would appear that they may be placed at a considerable disadvantage in future relationships, and may develop a variety of psychosexual problems that may both hinder the formation of a relationship or harm an existing one.

> It wasn't so bad before the colposcopy: I suppose I kept hoping it could be a mistake, maybe there was nothing wrong with me after all. But once the doctor said he could see an abnormal area on my cervix I knew it was true. I went home and cried. I didn't have a boyfriend, he'd cheated on me and we'd split up the year before. I felt really sorry for myself. No-one would ever want me now, I was dirty, maybe I was infectious, I had a disease. I felt like a leper. When I split up with Joe, I was angry, I knew he'd mistreated me. Suddenly I felt, maybe he'd been right, I was worthless.

These women and their partners need help. In recognition of this, some colposcopy units have set up counselling services, but they are still in a minority. It could be argued that counselling should become a routine part of the whole treatment process: prevention is better than cure.

More doctors are now aware of the problem and themselves try to make gentle enquiries as to how things are going. Sometimes all that is needed is to clear up a misunderstanding or a lack of information. If the problem is deeper, specialised counselling will be needed. You will find some addresses at the back of this book, or your clinic or GP may be able to give you further advice. A women's support group may be another useful source of help and information: sharing feelings and realising that other people have them too, is often helpful.

> Peter didn't seem particularly concerned at first, but I noticed he became more reserved. He still touched me and kissed me, but he'd always make excuses so that we didn't actually have sex. After the treatment we were told not to, anyway, but the month went past and he made no moves. I was a bit embarrassed to talk about it, I was having trouble coming to terms with the whole thing myself anyway. By the time I went for my check-up this had been going on for months. Luckily, I saw the same doctor as before. I decided to mention it. She asked if Peter had come with me: he was sitting outside. She called him in and had a general chat with both of us, stressing how sex couldn't harm me and that very few women had problems again in their lives after treatment. Peter asked specifically about that again during the conversation, and then said he'd been so worried that he might make the condition come back by having sex with me. The reassurance did the trick.

Cancer

There can be few pieces of news which are worse to give or receive than a diagnosis of cancer. The person receiving it sees before them a bleak future of pain, suffering and, ultimately, death. The person giving it knows this and feels a mixture of sympathy, sorrow and guilt, as though it were somehow their fault and that it is in some way unfair that they themselves are healthy. The family of the affected person will also have feelings of guilt, of sorrow and of helplessness. Sometimes this helplessness turns into hostility directed at the person giving the news, or even towards the woman herself. A great deal of understanding on all sides is therefore required at such a difficult time.

> I felt helpless, devastated. I didn't know what to do, I heard the doctor say 'cancer' and I just froze. I couldn't think of anything to ask. I just sat there.

The only thing I could think about was: 'Who's going to look after Jimmy and Kim? I won't see them grow up, I won't see them go to school, get married, nothing.'

A great deal may be said at the time the diagnosis is given, but it is unlikely that you or your family would take much in. It is therefore important to have a second appointment, fairly soon after the first, at which the whole issue can be discussed again. By this time, it is likely that you will have plenty of questions to ask.

It is worth bearing in mind, if you find yourself in this unhappy position, that the doctor who sees you is only a human being. It is very unlikely he or she has had any training in counselling techniques; it is somehow expected that these will be 'picked up' on the way. The doctor may therefore be feeling very awkward and may not really know what to say or how to say it, despite wanting to be as sympathetic and helpful as possible. However, do not feel inhibited from asking questions: it is often easier in such situations for the doctor to answer questions than to try and think what you might want or need to know.

Once again, the association of cervical cancer with sex makes some women feel very guilty. This is often particularly marked in women who have had abortions or extra-marital affairs. They may feel they are being punished for what they have done 'wrong'. Young women who have not had children may feel both cheated and punished, and may have strong feelings of both guilt and resentment.

I was so angry with myself. I knew I should have gone for a smear earlier, but I just kept putting it off. Really, I had no one but myself to blame.

My husband was awful. He kept saying 'you silly woman, why didn't you have the smear done when you were supposed to? Now see what's happened.' I knew it was really that he was so upset, but he made it much worse for me.

Women who feel they have 'got what they deserve' often become deceptively good, compliant patients. It is as if they feel they may get a reprieve for good behaviour. This is a mistake, as deep feelings of anger, resentment and fear may be suppressed. Such bargaining is likely to lead only to disappointment and further psychological problems; counselling is a much better solution.

139

Hysterectomy

The treatment of cancer often requires a hysterectomy (removal of the womb, or uterus). Many women, even if they have completed their family, find this daunting and disturbing. The uterus is often perceived as the essence of a woman's femininity; without it she may feel she is no longer a 'complete' woman. Also, periods are sometimes felt to be a 'cleansing of the system', without which poisons of some kind will accumulate in the body.

> It felt strange, the idea of having my womb removed. In one way, the thought of not having periods and not needing contraception anymore was good; but more often I found it frightening.

What you have to remember is that the womb is nothing more than a box in which to hold a baby. It has no other function. The blood that is shed each month is only the lining of the womb, which has thickened during the cycle in preparation for a fertilised egg that never materialised. Periods have no other meaning or function.

> I thought 'My husband will start looking around, I'll be like an old woman.'

The ovaries are not usually removed, unless you are approaching the menopause anyway. Even if they are removed, you can use hormone replacement therapy (HRT). It is not possible to go into all the pros and cons of hormone replacement here: obviously, you will need to find out more for yourself – but do not dismiss it outright because of things you have read in the papers. Even short-term use can be helpful for many women and, if you are young, you should be aware that using HRT only 'adds back' the oestrogen your ovaries would have been producing anyway. The potential risks of HRT are only relevant to women who are, in effect, postponing their menopause by taking the hormones at a time when their body would not be producing them naturally.

Any type of hysterectomy involves a considerable change in a woman's self-image. For a start, she will no longer be capable of having children. There is a world of difference between 'I don't want any (or any more) children' and 'I can't have any (or any more) children'.

> It was a relief, really, not to worry about contraception any more. We've got two children and that's enough! I'd been wondering whether to have a sterilisation: this solved both problems at once.

I was devastated. True, we had two lovely boys and hadn't been trying for another child. But it had been in the back of my mind that it might be nice to have a little girl. Suddenly, the decision wasn't mine any more.

Some women find the idea of sex with no possibility of becoming pregnant difficult. All methods of contraception have a failure rate, no matter how small: this element of risk may be crucial for some women to enjoy sex. They may therefore lose interest in sex after a hysterectomy.

I was embarrassed. I thought maybe my husband would notice the difference inside when we had sex. I felt somehow like a freak, an abnormal woman. Although I looked normal to other people, I didn't feel normal myself.

I was so worried that sex would be no good that I didn't want to try. I thought the longer I could put it off, somehow maybe the problem would go away. My boyfriend was very understanding, but after 6 months he started suggesting we should talk about it, try it. I found it very hard.

Many women worry that they will not be able to have sex normally after their operation. This can, of course, become a self-fulfilling prophecy, as the anxiety interferes with their sexual desire, their enjoyment and so on.

In fact a hysterectomy should, in theory, make little or no difference to a woman's life, including her sex life. During the weeks following the operation you are bound to feel tired and weak. Many women say it takes 2, even 3 months before they feel themselves again. However, it is important to try and resume sexual activity sooner rather than later; the later you leave it, the more likely you are to experience difficulty when restarting. Don't feel a failure if you need to use lubricants: anxiety affects your lubrication, and you are bound to feel anxious at the start. If you allow this situation to become a vicious circle (anxiety, dryness, more anxiety, more dryness, etc.), you will not be doing yourself a favour. Perhaps just as importantly, your partner needs to understand that you are not dry due to lack of interest in him; it is the anxiety, uncertainty and embarrassment of your situation.

The role of a supportive partner cannot be emphasised enough. Several studies and surveys have shown that women in long-term stable relationships fare much better than single women or those in unstable relationships. Indeed, women who are young and not in a relationship generally find it very difficult to start a new relationship afterwards. A partner can do a great deal to allays fears of rejection, unattractiveness and loss of femininity. Even when actual intercourse is impossible, he can show his affection in other ways: this maintains a woman's confidence in herself and their relationship.

His reaction was 'It's your problem, I'm getting out' and that was it. He just left.

We'd been going through a bad patch and I suppose this was the last straw.

While a good relationship is positively helpful, an unstable one may collapse under the strain of illness and suffering. Similarly, women who tend towards depression and anxiety in normal life are more likely to suffer after the operation.

It was odd: I was so strong throughout all the treatment. Everyone remarked on how determined I was. And yet when they finally told me I was OK, I fell apart.

I'd given up everything else in my life to concentrate on surviving. It was my only goal. When I was told I was cured, I thought 'what do I do now?'

Sometimes, even being pronounced cured can be stressful. Having channelled every ounce of strength and emotion into coping with cancer, it can be difficult to readjust to being a normal, healthy person. Again, understanding from family and friends is important in making the adjustment successfully. Some women have found it helpful to run a support group for others, or help with one: passing on your experiences can be useful therapy for all concerned.

Radiotherapy

Many people are frightened of radiation and therefore fear this treatment almost as much as the disease itself. The fact that the treatment goes on for several weeks and is often accompanied by ill-health, does not help with coping with it emotionally. It is very important to have enough time to discuss your fears and worries about side effects with the consultant. Also, remember that although you will be told about the possible side effects, that does not mean you will necessarily get them.

Unfortunately, radiotherapy causes the tissues in the pelvis to stiffen or fibrose and this does often lead to problems during sex. Advice is needed as to positions that will be most comfortable: the most successful are likely to be those in which deep penetration does not occur, at least initially. Radiotherapy also interferes with the function of the ovaries, resulting in a lack of oestrogen. Again, hormone replacement therapy is very useful: not only does it help psychologically and symptomatically, but it actually helps in the healing of the tissues.

One of the side effects that occurs during treatment is that women may notice vaginal discharge and bleeding, especially after intercourse. This is particularly alarming, as these are likely to be the very symptoms that led to the diagnosis of cancer. It is important to understand that they are simply a side effect and not signs of things getting worse.

Some people think that they become dangerous to others while receiving radiotherapy, which may add to negative feelings they already have about themselves. It is only true, and then only for a short time, if a source of radiation is actually placed within the body. It certainly does not apply to external radiation treatment: you do not glow in the dark afterwards.

I wish they could just have done an operation: all this to-ing and fro-ing and never feeling well, it's wearing me down.

Radiotherapy is often viewed with disappointment when compared to surgery – it is nicer to feel that the cancer has been actually cut out and taken away. This is not the case with radiotherapy, but it is important to remember that it can still result in a cure.

Chemotherapy

Nowadays, radiotherapy is often combined with chemotherapy. Different drugs have different side effects, so you need to check what is likely to happen in your own specific case. In general, though, the most common problems are reduced resistance to infections, nausea, diarrhoea, hair loss, mouth ulcers and feeling tired. Most of these problems only last for the couple of days after you have had the drugs, and hair does grow back.

Finally

While reading this chapter, you may once or twice have thought 'surely sex is the last thing on any woman's mind when she is ill, may even have cancer?' That is certainly true initially, when a woman is mostly concentrating on fighting the illness and being cured. But 95% of women with CIN are cured after the first treatment. Even those unfortunate enough to have early cancer still have a reasonable chance of cure. Life then has to go on.

The association of cervical cancer with sex makes it almost inevitable that women will be thinking about sex and relationships, even if the physical side is not currently an issue. Indeed, you may start to review your whole attitude to life and love. Some women ultimately find it a positive experience:

> I sat down and thought about my life. What a waste, I was just drifting. I wasn't being stretched in my job, Peter and I had long just been coexisting. I hadn't faced up to any of these things. I think the feeling that I might die (even though rationally I knew I didn't have cancer) made me want to change my life, do something useful with it.

In March 1989, *The Lancet*, a leading medical journal, published excerpts from a letter it had received from a doctor who herself had had an abnormal smear. She had suffered a horrific experience, among many other things:

> The tone of grim satisfaction with which the clinic nurse told me 'that's what comes from sleeping with too many men too young' made me want to hit her.

Her examination was watched by nine or ten male observers:

> that gaggle of men's faces peering down my vagina is not a pleasant memory.

She concludes:

> the memory of the pain, embarrassment and trauma remains, and is re-activated whenever I have the smallest gynaecological problem.

Since then, there has been increasing recognition of the emotional toll on women with abnormal smears, CIN and cancer. Counselling, once unheard of, has been introduced into some colposcopy clinics. Lack of funding has limited the progress in this area, but awareness of it has increased nevertheless. Hopefully, your experience will be an improvement on those of some women in the past.

Some of the emotional difficulties experienced by women and their partners are due to a lack of information or a misunderstanding of the facts. By reading this book I hope you will at least manage to avoid those problems and will have gained some understanding of the emotional processes which may seem bewildering and frightening, but are not uncommon. You are not alone, and there are counsellors and support groups out there: help can be found if you ask.

11   LOOKING AHEAD – POSSIBILITIES FOR THE FUTURE

We have seen that, as it currently stands, the cervical smear is not perfect. It would be nice to have a simple, preferably automated test that was more accurate. During the last 15 years there has been an increasing amount of research aimed at improving cervical screening. Inevitably, there have been disappointments, 'breakthroughs' that turned out to be false hopes. This chapter discusses techniques and research that, at present, appear promising – but any one of them could yet fail to live up to expectations. If you have not read Chapter 8 yet, I would suggest you do so before you continue with this chapter, as many of the concepts referred to here are explained in that chapter.

Cervicography

Cervicography is one of those innovations that was thought to be 'it' for a while, but has waned. Cervicography is simply a technique for taking photographs of the cervix without using a colposcope. As previously mentioned, smears rely heavily on human input and are therefore subject to human error. If only every woman could have a colposcopy instead of a smear – but that is neither practical (the costs are enormously higher), nor would all women consider it acceptable.

Colpophotography is the name given to the technique of taking photographs through a colposcope. In this case, the camera relies on the lens within the colposcope itself, so it has to be physically attached to a colposcope. The gynaecologist who developed cervicography had trained as a photographer before doing medicine. He realised that what was needed was a simple technique that would enable photographs of the cervix to be taken without the need for a colposcope. What he developed was the cerviscope (see Figure 11.1).

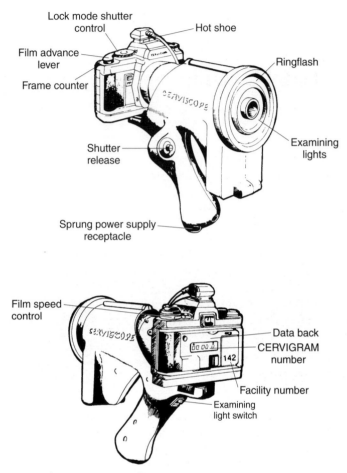

Film advance lever
Lock mode shutter control
Hot shoe
Frame counter
Ringflash
Shutter release
Examining lights
Sprung power supply receptacle

Film speed control
Data back
CERVIGRAM number
142
Facility number
Examining light switch

Figure 11.1   The components of a cerviscope.

He started out with an ordinary 35 mm SLR camera. A special lens was needed in order to allow photographs to be taken of a small object (i.e. the cervix), but without having the camera close: you wouldn't want the camera inside you, I'm sure! Then there was the problem of lighting; it is very dark looking down a speculum. For this reason, there is a powerful ring flash, as well as an ordinary light facility, so that the operator can see what he or she is doing. Everything possible has been fixed or automated, to make it as foolproof as possible.

148

A speculum is inserted and some dilute acetic acid is applied to the cervix just as in colposcopy. Then a photograph is taken and the procedure is repeated to obtain a second picture. Any doctor or nurse who takes smears can do cervicography. The photographs are of the whole cervix and are sent for evaluation to an expert in colposcopy. The evaluation (which includes an assessment of the estimated degree of abnormality) is then sent back to the clinic, together with a print that can be kept in the woman's records.

Cervicography misses very little, so false-negative results are not a problem. However, it has the opposite problem: it gives false-positive results. Even after a number of years of refinement, if a cervicogram is

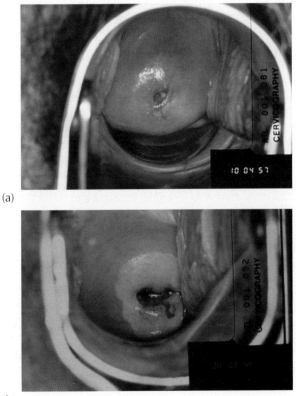

(a)

(b)

Figure 11.2 A couple of cervicograms: (a) normal, (b) abnormal.

149

reported as abnormal there is around a one in four chance it will turn out to be nothing. Why should this happen? In Chapter 4 I mentioned the problem that not everything which turns white with acetic acid is actually abnormal. This affects both colposcopy and cervicography. The doctor reporting the cervicogram sees an area that looks acetowhite, or abnormal: the only way to be sure is to take a biopsy, so it must be called 'positive'.

This problem with false-positive results is the main reason why cervicography is not suitable for mass screening programmes: the cost of the procedure, coupled with a partly unnecessary increase in workload for colposcopy clinics would overload the system and is not cost-effective. However, for an individual woman, it can be reassuring, and is used in some clinics in the USA. In the UK, very few doctors use it, and then mostly just for documentation and research.

Automated reading of cervical smears

Computerised smear reading is a real possibility. A computer can be programmed to recognise a large number of different cell appearances, and can be 'taught' which ones are normal and which suspicious. This eliminates a tedious feature of laboratory screening, which is that 90% of the samples checked are going to be normal. By using the computer system, cytologists only have to check those samples that are called suspicious. Although the equipment is expensive, it would potentially save time and manpower and, in addition, should reduce the laboratory false-negative rate.

HPV testing

In Chapter 8 we looked at the evidence for the involvement of HPV in cervical cancer. As we saw, there are 'high-risk' types, whose presence can help to predict which women have high grades of abnormality. Since HPV testing is discussed in detail in that chapter, I am only flagging it up here. The most likely use of HPV testing in the UK is for women who have a borderline smear. With the introduction of liquid-based cytology (see Chapter 1), it is possible to do an HPV test from the remainder of the stored sample, without the woman having to return for another examination. So, if a woman has a borderline smear, an HPV test could immediately be done in the laboratory: if it is positive she could be referred for colposcopy, whereas if it is negative, she could be reassured that it is safe to wait. There are studies being carried out in the UK looking at this issue and it is likely that a decision will be made in the next couple of years.

Molecular markers

As mentioned in Chapter 8, a problem with HPV testing is that it tends to give too many positive results, because it is not possible to tell a transient (harmless) from a persistent (potentially serious) infection. In the last few years, scientists have been looking at other proteins in cells, which may give a clue as to the stage of the HPV infection, and could be used in conjunction with HPV testing to improve its accuracy. These are still in the early stages and it is not possible to tell whether any of them will ultimately be useful, but it is a growing and interesting area of research.

Self-sampling for HPV

One of the problems with smear tests is that the examination involved is uncomfortable and women dislike having them done. The main problem is the use of the speculum, which is needed to allow the cervix to be seen and the sample taken from the right place (see Chapter 1). A good thing about HPV testing is that it isn't as dependent on getting cells from one

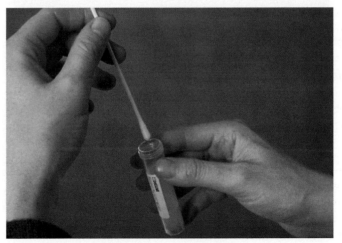

Figure 11.3 The cotton swab used for self-sampling.

particular place – if the infection is present, it will be spread over a large area. This opens up the possibility of women being able to test themselves, by just inserting a cotton swab into the vagina, in the privacy of their own homes. Studies have been carried out, comparing tests done by a doctor or nurse with those taken by women themselves, and the results are remarkably similar. So it may be that in the future you won't even need to go to a clinic, you will just do a test yourself at home. This may be particularly useful for women who really can't face the examination, and don't go for their smear test, but could be extended to all women. However, it will also depend on decisions made about how HPV testing should be used (see Chapter 8).

Electrical impedance probes (e.g. Polarprobe, TruScan)

This is a new concept in the field of cervical screening and diagnosis. It consists of a hand-held instrument which is inserted into the vagina and moved across the surface of the cervix. It uses a combination of

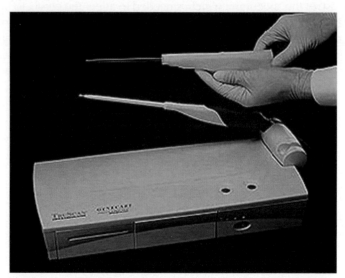

Figure 11.4   The TruScan probe. A plastic sheath, which is used only once and then discarded, fits over the TruScan probe. Photograph courtesy of CSIRO Mathematical and Information Sciences.

electrical pulses (but don't worry, you won't get an electric shock!) and low-intensity light to measure electrical activity and light reflections within cells. Scientists have shown that these are different in normal and abnormal cells. This information is relayed to a laptop computer, to which the probe is attached. Very sophisticated software has been designed so that the computer has an enormous database of normal and abnormal variants stored in its memory. When new signals come in, it rapidly compares them with the ones it knows and can thus give an assessment of the tissue. As you can imagine, this system depends on having every single possibility stored in its database, which is a major research activity and has now been ongoing for about 20 years. Recent studies suggest that the accuracy is improving, but there is still a little way to go.

If it fulfils its promise, there are several potential uses. It could be used in colposcopy, to give a more accurate assessment, instantly, of what degree of abnormality is present. As previously discussed, the white appearance that occurs with acetic acid does not always mean there is an abnormality. The probe could perhaps give an indication of the best place from which to take a biopsy, i.e. the place with the highest degree of abnormality.

The probe could be used in screening, if it were cheap enough. Every surgery and clinic would then have to have one, preferably one in each clinic room where women might be screened. The examination would then comprise the probe being inserted into the vagina and run over the surface of the cervix: presumably, great care would have to be taken not to miss any areas. An advantage would be the instant result. However, a disadvantage would be the lack of any documented evidence of the examination; if it was not carried out properly, there would presumably be no way of knowing. Such a careful examination of the cervix might necessitate the use of special couches, like those in colposcopy clinics. Also, rapid sterilisation of the probe between patients is an issue which is still not fully resolved (the most recent innovation has been to use a disposable plastic sheath for the device), but is clearly very important if it is to be used on a large scale.

Obviously, there are still details that need to be sorted out. However, this is an exciting idea which deserves further investigation.

More accessible colposcopy?

At present, there is a great shortage of gynaecologists trained in colposcopy. Clinics are overflowing with patients, waiting lists in some areas are several months long. Women are anxious while waiting to be seen and the whole situation is unsatisfactory. What can be done?

Of course, one solution would be to train more gynaecologists. But it is very unlikely that they would want to do nothing other than colposcopy, and then there might actually be overstaffing in other fields as a result. All this could become very expensive. Another alternative is to train up doctors who are not gynaecologists, but have had some gynaecological training. Such doctors could be GPs, family planning doctors and doctors working in sexual health clinics. Their advantage is that they are in any case likely to be dealing with women who have abnormal smears and are therefore both interested and experienced in this area. Colposcopy clinics have also realised the benefit of having doctors who come in for a few sessions a week, just to do colposcopy. These doctors often remain in the job for years, providing continuity and reducing the need to constantly train new junior doctors who are going to move on in 6 months or a year.

More recently, nurses have started to train as colposcopists and a growing number of nurse colposcopists are proving invaluable in colposcopy clinics around the country. Again, nurses are less likely to move on; also, women often find it easier to talk to a nurse, so they may find the examination less stressful. This is a trend that is set to continue, with some nurse colposcopists going on to learn how to perform loop diathermy treatments as well.

Vaccines

As we have seen, a number of human papillomavirus (HPV) types appear to be the main cause of cervical cancer. We have vaccines to protect us from other virus infections, for example, rubella (German measles) and smallpox. Why should we not be able to apply the same principle to cervical cancer?

A major problem in the development of a vaccine has been that HPV seems to be a particularly difficult virus to grow artificially: it only likes to reproduce in living cells and does not respond well to laboratory cell cultures. This means it has been difficult to produce enough of it for research studies, let alone start a production line for a vaccine. Also, there were worries about using the actual virus to produce a vaccine – there would always be the danger that the vaccine itself might cause disease in people whose immune system was deficient, as has occasionally happened, for example, with the polio vaccine.

The solution has been to manufacture virus-like particles (VLPs) using the virus coat proteins (see Figure 11.5). The DNA (deoxyribonucleic acid) of the virus is held inside a 'coat' or shell, made of two proteins, called L1 and L2. DNA is genetic material which is used by the virus to take control of a cell and make it do whatever it wants (see also Chapter 8). VLPs look like the actual virus, because they are made of the coat proteins, but they are harmless as they contain no DNA. However, because the body can't tell there is no virus inside, it mounts a powerful immune antibody response to the VLPs.

Another potential challenge has been the number of cervical cancer HPV types which need to be included (potentially 15). However, in practice, two HPV types, 16 and 18, actually cause 70% of cervical cancers, so those are the most important ones (see Figure 11.6). A vaccine that only protects against those two HPV types could prevent 70% of cervical cancers. If a couple more types could be included (or if cross-protection against other HPV types is confirmed, see below), the protection rate could go up to over 80%.

There are two HPV vaccines that have shown great promise. One of these (called Gardasil), which has recently been licensed, contains four

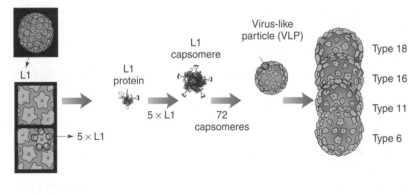

<figure>

L1

5 × L1

L1
protein

5 × L1

L1
capsomere

72
capsomeres

Virus-like
particle (VLP)

Type 18

Type 16

Type 11

Type 6

HPV virus:
L1 = external protein

HPV VLP vaccine

</figure>

Figure 11.5 The vaccine mimics the virus shell. Modified from an image kindly supplied by Sanofi Pasteur MSD.

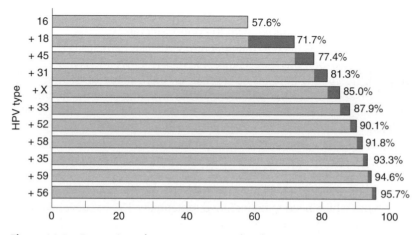

Figure 11.6 Proportion of cancers associated with HPV types.

HPV types, 6,11, 16 and 18, and would thus protect against genital warts (types 6 and 11) as well as the commonest cervical cancer HPV types (16 and 18). The other (called Cervarix, which is likely to be licensed in Summer 2007) contains types 16 and 18, and thus targets cervical cancer alone. Both vaccines have been tested in large, ongoing, multicentre, worldwide phase III clinical trials, and have been shown to be extremely effective, safe and well tolerated. (Phase III clinical trials are the last testing stage before a medication is given a licence. This means they have already been tested over many years in thousands of people.) Both vaccines appear to be 90–100% effective in preventing HPV infection in the first place (known as 'incident' infection) and also in preventing HPV infections from becoming persistent. (You will recall from Chapter 8 that it is persistent HPV infection with high-risk HPV types that is the problem.)

An interesting feature of HPV infection is that the virus is very successful at avoiding our immune system, and therefore causing natural immunity. I'm sure you know that if you catch, say, measles as a child, you are very unlikely ever to get it again, because you will have become immune. Unfortunately, this doesn't happen with HPV: it manages to 'hide' from the immune system and so you can get it again. However, both the HPV vaccines also contain an extra substance called an adjuvant (each of the vaccines has a different one). This stimulates the immune response and, because it is being given at the same time as the vaccine, results in the immune response to the vaccine itself being much stronger than it would have been otherwise. Studies have shown that the vaccines can produce antibody levels that are enormously (60 to 100 times) higher and longer lasting than those generated by natural infection.

A vaccine against cervical cancer is a very exciting prospect, but there are still a number of unanswered questions. Will there be any cross-protection against HPV types not included in the vaccines? This has always been thought unlikely, but in a recent study, a vaccine against types 16 and 18 also stimulated antibodies against other HPV types, including the high-risk types 31 and 45. This is potentially extremely important, as it may significantly raise the overall protection level.

If we eliminate cancer due to HPV types 16 and 18, will other HPV types take their place? It is thought unlikely but we don't have proof. Will we need different vaccines for different populations? Types 16 and 18 seem to be the most common types around the world, so hopefully not. What might be the effect of a vaccine in HIV-positive women? We don't know, studies are only just beginning in this area.

A tricky issue is deciding at which age it should be given, since it would be best to give it before the onset of sexual activity. In any case, for all vaccines, the immune response is better the earlier they are given – one of the reasons we have most of our vaccines in early childhood. The same has been shown to be true in this case – adolescents between 9 and 14 years had the strongest response. However, we do not know at present how long the immunity conferred by these vaccines lasts; the studies so far have shown efficacy up to 5 years. Ideally, the vaccine would be administered with other childhood vaccines, which would also remove any link with sexual activity in the minds of parents. However, that would depend on the immunity lasting for decades, or boosters being given. It is thought (based on the results so far, and extrapolating from information from other vaccines) that the immunity will last at least 10 years.

Should we not vaccinate boys as well as girls? Currently, there is interest only in vaccinating girls, mainly for financial reasons. There have also been fewer studies of the vaccines in boys, though they are ongoing and so far show that the immune response is also good in boys and men between the ages of 10 and 26. (It is important to show efficacy in both sexes, as, to use a recent example, a vaccine against the herpes virus was found to work in women but not in men.) In my view, concentrating wholly on women is a short-sighted and potentially damaging strategy. The rubella vaccination programme has provided evidence of the benefit of vaccinating both sexes despite the infection being of most importance in women. In Sweden the programme (as in many places) began only with girls. However, it was found to be only partially effective and rubella syndrome was only eradicated when both boys and girls were included in the programme. It is very unlikely that uptake of the vaccine by girls will even approach 100%, thus for so-called population or 'herd' immunity to develop, both boys and girls will need to be vaccinated. In addition, vaccination only of girls will ignore the needs of homosexual men, who are at higher than average risk of anal cancer (also mainly caused by HPV types 16 and 18) and genital warts. As yet, there have not been any studies carried out in this group, but there is clearly a need.

Studies, mainly of white, Afro-Caribbean or Hispanic people in North and South America, have found generally positive responses to the vaccine and a willingness to allow young girls to be vaccinated. However, vaccinating only girls has the effect of focusing attention on women in relation to a sexually transmitted virus; there are some cultures in which this may prove unacceptable. In those communities the role and sexual behaviour of men as vectors is ignored, but it would only be by vaccinating men that women could be protected. The vaccine, which contains the types causing genital warts as well as cervical cancer, may be the solution in such societies, as it could be presented as primarily protecting men from warts. Once again, a fundamental problem is the lack of education, of both the general public and doctors and nurses, about HPV.

In developing countries, where screening is often not available, HPV vaccination represents a great hope in the fight against cervical cancer. For a vaccination programme – in any country – to work, the acceptability and uptake of the vaccine is as important as its efficacy, so investigating attitudes to the vaccine and likely uptake are crucial.

As always, it is the developed countries that will have the earliest benefit from the preventive vaccines. Preliminary estimates suggest that the three injection course will cost around £200 for the vaccine alone, which is clearly unaffordable in poor countries. However, organisations such as the Alliance for Cervical Cancer Prevention, the World Health Organization and the Bill and Melinda Gates Foundation have all contributed to developing world projects, and could choose to help these countries set up vaccination programmes.

158

In theory, an HPV vaccine could prevent almost all cervical cancer, eventually removing the need for cervical smears. However, until the number of HPV types in the vaccine is increased, there will still be cancers not prevented by vaccination. In addition, there is at least one whole generation of women for whom it is likely that the vaccine will come too late, and who will continue to require screening. Studies are under way looking at whether the vaccines work in older (over 25 years old) women, who presumably have already been exposed to HPV. However, even if a woman has come in contact with one HPV type, the vaccines should still protect against other types to which she has not been exposed. We already know that women of all ages (up to 55) produce a good immune response to the HPV 16/18 vaccine. If the vaccines are shown to work in this older age group, this would have a much more immediate impact on cervical cancer rates. Exciting times lie ahead!

At the time of writing, the quadrivalent vaccine (against all four HPV types), Gardasil, has been licensed in many countries, including the UK, for use between the ages of 9 and 26 years. In the USA, a state vaccination programme is to be implemented for girls 11–12 years old. A decision regarding a vaccination programme is still awaited in the UK.

The bivalent vaccine (against types HPV 16 and 18) is called Cervarix and is likely to be licensed in the summer of 2007.

Therapeutic (treatment) vaccines

So far, I have only discussed vaccines which prevent HPV infection happening, or becoming persistent. There is another group of vaccines being studied, which might be able to reverse the abnormal cell changes and 'cure' women who already have an abnormality. However, these vaccines have been even more difficult to develop and are still in very early trials. We are not likely to see them in use for many years yet.

Finally

This is an exciting time in the field of cervical screening and colposcopy. There are a number of new ideas that really seem to be promising and we now have two preventive HPV vaccines. However, do not forget that the tried and tested, boring old cervical smear will still give you protection against cervical cancer – so make sure you go for yours.

FURTHER READING

This section provides details of studies or reference material for those who want to look up something specific. It is by no means comprehensive, but just a pointer to some papers of interest.

Chapter 2   What is an abnormal smear?

French DP, Maissi E, Marteau TM. Psychological costs of inadequate cervical smear test results. *Br J Cancer* 2004; **91**: 1887–1892.

Marteau TM, Walker P, Giles J, Smail M. Anxieties in women undergoing colposcopy. *Br J Obstet Gynaecol* 1990; **97(9)**: 859–861.

NHSCSP. *Colposcopy and Programme Management: Guidelines for the NHS Cervical Screening Programme.* NHSCSP Publication No. 20. Published April 2004. ISBN 1 84 4630 14 5. Available from http://cancerscreening.org.uk/cervical/publications.

Shafi MI, Luesley DM, Jordan JA, Dunn JA, Rollason TP, Yates M. Randomised trial of immediate versus deferred treatment strategies for the management of minor cervical cytological abnormalities. *Br J Obstet Gynaecol* 1997; **104(5)**: 590–594.

Chapter 3   What does this mean? A look at some technical terms

Martin-Hirsch P, Lilford R, Jarvis G, Kitchener HC. Efficacy of cervical-smear collection devices: a systematic review and meta-analysis. *Lancet* 1999; **354**: 1763–1770.

Chapter 4   Having a colposcopy examination

NHSCSP. *Colposcopy and Programme Management: Guidelines for the NHS Cervical Screening Programme.* NHSCSP Publication No. 20. Published April

161

2004. ISBN 1 84 4630 14 5. Available from http://cancerscreening.org.uk/cervical/publications.

Chapter 5   Treatment options for CIN

http://www.cancerhelp.co.uk/help/default.asp?page=2739.

Chapter 6   Cervical cancer and its treatment

http://www.cancerhelp.co.uk/help/default.asp?page=2739.

Chapter 7   Why me? The possible causes of CIN and cervical cancer

Bosch FX, Iftner T. The aetiology of cervical cancer. NHSCSP Publication No. 22. ISBN 1 84 4630 23 4. Published September 2005. Available from http://cancerscreening.org.uk/cervical/publications/nhscsp22.html.

La Vecchia C, Franceschi S, Decarli A, Fasoli M, Gentile A, Tognoni G. Cigarette smoking and the risk of cervical neoplasia. *Am J Epidemiol* 1986; **123**: 22–29.

Szarewski A, Cuzick J. Smoking and cervical cancer: a review of the evidence. *J Epidemiol Biostats* 1998; **3(3)**: 229–256.

Szarewski A, Jarvis MJ, Sasieni P, *et al.* The effect of smoking cessation on cervical lesion size. *Lancet* 1996; **347**: 941–943.

Chapter 8   The role of viruses

Kjaer SK, van den Brule AJ, Bock JE, *et al.* Human papillomavirus – the most significant risk determinant of cervical intraepithelial neoplasia. *Int J Cancer* 1996; **65(5)**: 601–606.

Koutsky L. Epidemiology of genital human papillomavirus infection. *Am J Med.* 1997; **102(5A)**: 3–8.

Walboomers JM, Jacobs MV, Manos MM, *et al.* Human papillomavirus is a necessary cause of invasive cervical cancer worldwide. *J Pathol* 1999; **189**:12–19.

Chapter 9   The cervical screening controversy: how often should you have a smear?

NHSCSP. *Colposcopy and Programme Management: Guidelines for the NHS Cervical Screening Programme.* NHSCSP Publication No. 20. Published April 2004. ISBN 1 84 4630 14 5. Available from http://cancerscreening.org.uk/cervical/publications.

Sasieni P, Adams J. Effect of screening on cervical cancer mortality in England and Wales: analysis of trends with an age period cohort model. *Br Med J* 1999; **318**: 1244–1245.

Sasieni P, Adams J, Cuzick J. Benefits of cervical screening at different ages: evidence from the UK audit of screening histories. *Br J Cancer* 2003; **89**: 88–93.

Chapter 10   Emotional feelings and reactions

French DP, Maissi E, Marteau TM. Psychological costs of inadequate cervical smear test results. *Br J Cancer* 2004; **91**: 1887–1892.

Maissi E, Marteau TM, Hankins M, Moss S, Legood R, Gray A. Psychological impact of human papillomavirus testing in women with borderline or mildly dyskaryotic cervical smear test results: cross-sectional questionnaire study. *Br Med J* 2004; **328**: 1293.

Marteau TM, Walker P, Giles J, Smail M. Anxieties in women undergoing colposcopy. *Br J Obstet Gynaecol* 1990; **97(9)**: 859–861.

McCaffery K, Irwig L. Australian women's needs and preferences for information about human papillomavirus in cervical screening. *J Med Screen* 2005; **12**: 134–141.

McCaffery KJ, Forrest S, Waller J, Desai M, Szarewski A, Wardle J. Attitudes towards HPV testing: a qualitative study of beliefs among Indian, Pakistani, African Caribbean and white British women in the UK. *Br J Cancer* 2003; **88**: 42–46.

McCaffery KJ, Waller J, Forrest S, Cadman L, Szarewski A, Wardle J. Testing positive for human papillomavirus in routine cervical screening: examination of the psychosocial impact. *Br J Obstet Gynaecol* 2004; **111**: 1437–1443.

Waller J, McCaffery K, Wardle J. Beliefs about the risk factors for cervical cancer in a British population sample. *Prev Med* 2004; **38**: 745–753.

Waller J, McCaffery KJ, Forrest S, Szarewski A, Cadman L, Wardle J. Awareness of human papillomavirus (HPV) among women attending a well woman clinic. *Sex Transm Infect* 2003; **79**: 320–322.

Chapter 11   Looking ahead – possibilities for the future

Bottiger M, Forsgren M. Twenty years' experience of rubella vaccination in Sweden: 10 years of selective vaccination (of 12-year-old girls and of women postpartum) and 13 years of a general two-dose vaccination. *Vaccine* 1997; **15(14)**:1538–1544.

Garland SM, Hernandez-Avila M, Wheeler CM, *et al.* Quadrivalent vaccine against human papillomavirus to prevent anogenital disesaes. *N Engl J Med* 2007; **356**: 1928–1943.

Harper DM, Franco EL, Wheeler CM, *et al*. Sustained efficacy up to 4.5 years of a bivalent L1 virus-like particle vaccine against human papillomavirus types 16 and 18: follow-up from a randomised control trial. *Lancet* 2006; **367**: 1247–1255.

Joura E, Leodotter S, Hernandez-Avila M, *et al*. Efficacy of a quadrivalent prophylactic human papillomavirus (types 6, 11, 16 and 18) L1 virus-like-particle vaccine against high-grade vulval and vaginal lesions: a combined analysis of three randomised clinical trials. *Lancet* 2007; **369**: 1693–1702.

Koutsky L, *et al*. The Future II Study Group. Quadrivalent HPV vaccine against human papillomavirus to prevent high-grade cervical lesions. *N Engl J Med* 2007; **356**: 1915–1927.

Stanley MA. Human papillomavirus (HPV) vaccines: prospects for eradicating cervical cancer. *J Fam Plann Reprod Health Care* 2004; **30(4)**: 213–217.

Szarewski A. Prophylactic vaccines for HPV: a bright future for cervical cancer prevention. *J Med Screen* 2005; **12**: 163–165.

Villa LL, Costa RR, Petta CA, *et al*. Prophylactic quadrivalent human papillomavirus (types 6, 11, 16 and 18) L1 virus-like particle vaccine in young women: a randomised double-blind placebo controlled multicentre phase II efficacy trial. *Lancet Oncol* 2005; **6 (5)**: 271–278.

USEFUL ADDRESSES

UK

The NHS Cervical Screening Programme

This is the organisation that actually runs the cervical screening programme. They have a useful website and produce information leaflets.

National coordination office

NHS Cancer Screening Programmes
The Manor House
260 Ecclesall Road South
Sheffield S11 9PS
Telephone: 0114 271 1060/1
Fax: 0114 271 1089
Website: www.cancerscreening.nhs.uk

Public relations and press enquiries

NHS Cancer Screening Programmes press office
3 London Wall Buildings
London Wall
London EC2M 5SY
Telephone: 020 7282 2922
Fax: 020 7282 1064
Email: screening@westminster.com

NHS Direct

This is a 24-hour phone line for medical queries.
Telephone: 0845 4647

European Cervical Cancer Association (ECCA)

Website: http://www.ecca.info/webECCA/en/
The website has been specifically set up to provide information for the public about cervical cancer, screening and HPV. It also provides links to other sites and to relevant scientific papers.

Cancer charities

Cancer Research UK

PO Box 123
Lincoln's Inn Fields
London WC2A 3PX
Telephone: 020 7242 0200
Website: http://www.cancerresearchuk.org
Email: cancerhelpuk@cancer.org.uk

Cancer Research UK Information Nurses

Cancer Research UK was formed from the merger of The Cancer Research Campaign and The Imperial Cancer Research Fund. It is the foremost cancer charity in the UK and the largest cancer research organisation in the world, outside the USA. It funds doctors and scientists in hospitals, medical schools, universities and research institutes across the UK. Cancer Research UK is the European leader in the development of new anti-cancer drugs. It funds research on all aspects of the disease from its causes to treatment and prevention, education and psychological support for patients. Cancer Research UK also supports the CancerHelp UK website and is responsible for developing and maintaining the site's Clinical Trials Database.
Email: cancer.info@cancer.org.uk
Telephone: 020 7061 8355

Action Cancer

1 Marlborough Place
Belfast BT9 6HQ
Telephone: 028 9066 1081
Fax: 028 9068 3931
    Action Cancer is a local charity committed to fighting breast cancer and cervical cancer since 1978. Action Cancer has a full-time clinic and

166

mobile unit for early detection and screening and offers one-to-one counselling. Services are free. Action Cancer also funds a leading research team at Queen's University, Belfast.

British Association for Counselling and Psychotherapy
BACP House
35–37 Albert Street
Rugby
Warks CV21 2SG
Telephone: 0870 443 5252
Website: www.bacp.co.uk
    This organisation produces a directory of qualified counsellors and psychotherapists. The directory is updated each year. They can provide you with a list of counsellors in your area. You can search online, phone for information or their directory may be available in your local library.

CancerBACUP
3 Bath Place
Rivington Street
London EC2A 3JR
Freephone: 0808 800 1234
Admin: 020 7696 9003
Fax: 020 7696 9002
Website: www.cancerbacup.org.uk

CancerBACUP Scotland
3rd floor, Cranston House
104–114 Argyle Street
Glasgow G2 8BH
Freephone helpline: 0808 800 1234
    CancerBACUP – the British Association of Cancer United Patients. This charity was founded by Dr Vicky Clement-Jones after her own experiences with cancer. CancerBACUP offers information, advice and emotional support to cancer patients and their families. It has publications about the main types of cancer, treatments and ways of living with cancer. CancerBACUP also produces a newsletter, CancerBACUP News. There is also a freephone telephone and letter information service, provided by a team of specialist cancer nurses, on all aspects of cancer and treatment and walk-in centres at six hospitals around the country.

167

The Ulster Cancer Foundation
Villa 2
Belvoir Park Hospital
Hospital Road
Belfast BT8 3JR
Telephone helpline: 0800 783 33 39
Admin: 028 9049 2007
Website: www.ulstercancer.org
Email: ucf.info@ulstercancer.org
   Provides a cancer information helpline, information and resource cen-
tre, public and professional education. Rehabilitation programmes and
support groups for patients and relatives.

Women's Health Concern
PO Box 2126
Marlow
Bucks SL7 2RY
Telephone helpline: 0845 123 2319
Website: www.womens-health-concern.org
   Organisation that provides information about many women's health
issues. Can give personalised advice on menopause problems and hor-
mone replacement therapy. Professional counselling available. Produces
booklets on a range of subjects including hormone replacement therapy,
menopause, hysterectomy and ovarian cysts. WHC nurses provide a serv-
ice from Monday to Friday, 9 a.m.–5 p.m.

Women's Nationwide Cancer Control Campaign
1st Floor
Charity House
14–15 Perseverance Works
London E2 8DD
Telephone: 020 7729 4688 (General Enquiries)
Fax: 020 7613 0771
   This is a national cancer charity for women dedicated to promoting
the prevention and early detection of cancers affecting women. It emphasises the importance of cervical smears and breast awareness, encour-
ages healthy living, and promotes and facilitates the participation of
women in the NHS breast and cervical screening programmes.

168

Services include:

- providing health talks and information at public meetings, workplaces and exhibitions;
- producing a range of health education materials to answer common questions about cancer prevention and screening;
- working to encourage women to take part in screening, particularly those from low-uptake groups.

Jo's Trust
Weedon Villa
Everdon
Northamptonshire NN11 3BQ
Email: pamela@jotrust.co.uk
Telephone: +44 (0) 1327 341965
Fax: +44 (0) 1327 349397
Website: http://www.jotrust.co.uk/

Jo's Trust is a registered charity dedicated to women with cervical cancer. Its primary activity is an online cervical cancer information, confidential medical advice and counselling service. Its secondary aim is to raise the public profile and understanding of cervical cancer and how it can be beaten.

Other organisations

Relate
Central Office: Herbert Gray College
Little Church Street
Rugby CV21 3AP
Telephone helpline: 0845 130 40 10
Website: www.relate.org.uk

Nationwide network of clinics providing private and confidential counselling, and psychosexual therapy to help with relationship problems. Local branches can be found in telephone directories.

British Association for Sexual and Relationship Therapy
PO Box 13686
London SW20 9ZH

Telephone: 020 8543 2707
Website: www.basrt.org.uk
Provides information about what help and therapy is available for sexual difficulties.

Sexual Dysfunction Association
Windmill Place Business Centre
2–4 Windmill Lane
Southall UB2 4NJ
Telephone: 0870 774 3571
Website: www.sda.uk.net
Information on sexual problems that can affect men and women. They provide lists of local specialist practitioners, as well as factsheets on problems such as errectile dysfunction (impotence).

The Family Planning Association
Gives advice on all aspects of family planning, sexual problems, etc. A good source of information about other clinics and services available throughout the United Kingdom. They produce leaflets on many topics.

England
2–12 Pentonville Road
London N1 9FP
Telephone helpline: the low-cost national helpline number is 0845 310 1334 (Monday to Friday 9 a.m.–6 p.m.)
Telephone: 020 7837 5432
Fax: 0845 123 2349

Northern Ireland
Belfast
113 University Street
Belfast BT7 1HP
Telephone helpline: 028 9032 5488 (Monday to Thursday 9 a.m.–5 p.m., Friday 9 a.m.–4.30 p.m.)
Fax: 028 9031 2212

Derry
2nd Floor, Northern Counties Building
Custom House Street

Derry BT48 6AE
Telephone helpline: 028 7126 0016 (Monday to Thursday 9 a.m.–5 p.m.,
Friday 9 a.m.–4.30 p.m.)
Fax: 028 7136 1254

Scotland
Glasgow
Unit 10, Firhill Business Centre
76 Firhill Road
Glasgow G20 7BA
Telephone helpline: 0141 576 5088 (Monday to Thursday 9 a.m.–5 p.m.,
Friday 9 a.m.–4.30 p.m.)
Telephone: 0141 948 1170
Fax: 0141 948 1172

Wales
Cardiff
Suite D1, Canton House
435–451 Cowbridge Road East
Cardiff CF5 1JH
Telephone: 029 2064 4034
Fax: 029 2064 4306

Bangor
Greenhouse
Trevelyan Terrace
Bangor
Gwynedd LL57 1AX
Telephone: 01248 353 534
Fax: 01248 371 138

Brook
Head Office
421 Highgate Studios
53–79 Highgate Road
London NW5 1TL
Telephone helpline: 0800 0185 023 (Monday to Friday, 9 a.m.–5 p.m.)
Telephone: 020 7284 6040

Fax: 020 7284 6050
Email: www.brook.org.uk
Nationwide network of clinics. Specialise in young people's problems (under 25). Provide family planning, screening services and counselling

Terence Higgins Trust
52–54 Grays Inn Road
London WC1X 8JU
Telephone: 020 7831 0330
Fax: 020 7242 0121
Email: info@tht.org.uk
Website: www.tht.org.uk
Information, support groups and counselling about AIDS.

The Herpes Association
41 North Road
London N7 9DP
Telephone: 0845 123 2305
Email: info@herpes.org.uk
Website: www.herpes.org.uk/
Information and support for people with herpes.

ASH Action on Smoking and Health
102 Clifton Street
London EC2A 4HW
Telephone: +44 (0)20 7739 5902
Fax: +44 (0)20 7613 0531
Email: enquiries@ash.org.uk
Website: http://www.ash.org.uk
Advice on stopping smoking and wider issues to do with tobacco control.

The Hysterectomy Support Network
3 Lynne Close
Green Street Green
Orpington

172

Kent BR6 6BS
Telephone: 020 8856 3881
Refers women (and family or partners) concerned about hysterectomy to former patients in their area, who will provide encouragement, advice and support through the informal sharing of experiences and information. Booklet and information about membership of local support groups available. Contact by letter, or through group meetings

Private Family Planning Clinics

Marie Stopes House
The Well Woman Centre
108 Whitfield Street
London W1P 5RU
Telephone: 071 388 0662/2585

Marie Stopes Centre
10 Queen Square
Leeds LS2 8AJ
Telephone: 0532 440685

Marie Stopes Centre
1, Police Street
Manchester M2 7LQ
Telephone: 061 832 4250
Cervical screening, HPV testing and colposcopy are available at the Marie Stopes Clinics.

Eire

Irish Family Planning Clinic
Cathal Brugha Street Clinic
Dublin 1
Telephone: Dublin 727276/727363
Provides a similar service to the FPA within the confines of Irish law.

USA

Planned Parenthood Federation of America
Head office
2010 Massachusetts Avenue
NW Suite 500
Washington DC 20036
Telephone: 202 785 3351

Western region
333 Broadway
3rd Floor
San Francisco
CA 94133
Telephone: 415 956 8856

Southern region
3030 Peachtree Road
NW Room 303
Atlanta
GA 30305

Northern region
2625 Butterfield Rd
Oak Brook
IL 60521
Telephone: 312 986 9270

Australia

Australian Federation of FPAs
Suite 603
6th floor
Roden Cutler House
24 Campbell Street
Sydney
NSW 2000

New Zealand

The New Zealand FPA Inc.
PO Box 68200
214 Karangahape
Newton
Auckland

South Africa

FPA of South Africa
412 York House
46 Kerk Street
Johannesburg 2001

INDEX

ibuprofen 61, 62, 64
imiquimod 110
immune cells 79–80, 94
immune response to viruses 100–101
immune system 37, 128
  deficiencies 97–98, 106–107
  human papillomavirus 106–108,
    156–157
  pregnancy 98
infections
  abnormal smears 36–43
  cervical smear 15
  microscopic 130
  see also herpes simplex virus (HSV);
    human papillomavirus (HPV); viral
    infections
inflammatory changes, severe 44–45
information
  about abnormal smears 22–23
  about human papillomavirus 133
internal os 2, 3
  cone biopsy 71–72
intrauterine contraceptive device (IUD)
    13–14
  actinomyces-like organisms 42, 43
  laser vaporisation/loop diathermy
    64–65
intravenous pyelogram 83
iodine 50–51

Jewish people 90, 91, 93

kidneys, examination 83
koilocytes 105

lactic acid 37
lactobacillus 37
Langerhans cells 94
laser vaporisation 57–59, 61–65
  care after 63–64
  colposcopy after 65
  cone biopsy 73
  IUDs 64–65
leaflets about abnormal smears 22–23
liquid-based cytology (LBC) 10, 29–30, 131
  human papillomavirus testing 112, 113

local anaesthetic 62–63
loop diathermy 28, 57, 59–65
  care after 63–64
  colposcopy after 65
  cone biopsy 73
  IUDs 64–65
  long-term problems 65
  specimen for examination 59–60
  treatment failure 65
lymph channels 79–80
lymph nodes, removal 84, 85
lymphangiogram 83–84

magnetic resonance imaging (MRI) 84
mefenamic acid 61, 62, 64
men
  high-risk 91
  human papillomavirus 93, 108
  reaction to abnormal smear results
    131–132
  reaction to cancer diagnosis 139, 142
  reaction to colposcopy and treatment
    137, 138
  sexual behaviour 90–91, 128
  support after HPV diagnosis 130–131
  support after hysterectomy 141–142
menopause 128
  oestrogen levels 45
menstrual bleeding
  laser/loop diathermy treatment 61–62
  postponing 62
menstrual cycle
  appearance of cells 13
  taking smears 9–10
metronidazole 40, 42
miscarriage 72
molecular markers 151
monilia 36

Nabothian follicles 5
NHS Cervical Screening Programme 25
nicotine 93–94
Nurofen 61, 62, 64
nurses 49
  colposcopy training 154
nystatin 38

181